Explaining Parkinson's

Contents

Introduction

A good deal has been written about Parkinson's over the years, and there are many avenues through which information about the condition can be obtained. Throughout this book, which has been revised and updated as a third edition to include findings new to Parkinson's and also rights in the workplace, I will be also referring to various organisations that play a major role in providing invaluable information about Parkinson's disease.

My own background is non-medical so it should be understood from the outset that what you read in this book is in no way based on medical opinion, it is just a product of research and personal experiences. My personal experiences have involved my partner's relatives and very close friends of mine and I have been deeply involved in all aspects of Parkinson's from initial diagnosis to living with Parkinson's and medication and ongoing needs and support.

In addition to this, I myself was diagnosed mistakenly with Parkinson's disease by my doctor (although I hasten to add this was an initial diagnosis and he referred me to a specialist who, after a few months of tests, and a deep brain scan, informed me that I did not in fact have Parkinson's). What this little episode did was take me through the initial phase of trauma and then acceptance that I might have Parkinson's disease. It was the culmination of all these experiences that prompted me, with the aid of my partner, to write this book.

What is Parkinson's?

Parkinson's is (one of) the most common disorders of the nervous system. Muscle movements are affected with the main symptoms being tremors, stiffening of the muscles and, overall, slower movement patterns. Parkinson's was first identified in 1817 by Doctor James Parkinson, working in London. Although the condition has been in existence for a very long time, it is now more prevalent because of the aging population, the fact that people are living longer. It is recognised most frequently in people of 60 or over, although it is also prevalent in some younger people.

Doctors are now far more aware of Parkinson's and the advances in drugs available to treat them have been very significant, particularly in the last decade. Research nowadays is focussed on slowing and preventing the progression of the condition and there will be corresponding advances in the types of medication available.

This brief book covers the diagnosis of Parkinson's, dealing with the condition in its early stages and explaining the condition to others, choosing the most effective medication for you, choosing diet and putting together an exercise regime, a discussion of surgical options and also the financial aspects of Parkinson's such as benefits and employment. There is a section about people who care for those with Parkinson's and many useful contacts.

Initially, a lot of medical terminology is used and I do my best to elaborate on the meanings of various terms. I sincerely hope that you will benefit from this brief but nonetheless important and informative book .

Doreen Jarrett 2016

Chapter 1
The Underlying Causes of Parkinson's

As was mentioned in the introduction, Parkinson's was identified almost 200 years ago. However, as with a lot of illnesses, the exact cause of the condition remains a mystery, notwithstanding lots of research, and a number of factors are seen as contributory.

The brain

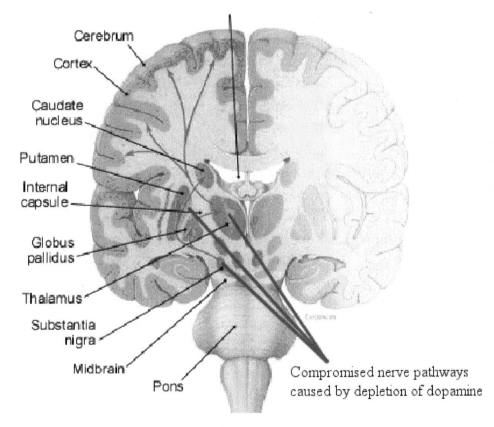

Cerebrum
Cortex
Caudate nucleus
Putamen
Internal capsule
Globus pallidus
Thalamus
Substantia nigra
Midbrain
Pons

Compromised nerve pathways caused by depletion of dopamine

The root of Parkinson's lies within the brain. Obviously, it is very difficult to treat the brain in a mechanistic way as it incorporates our mind and is our very existence. However, scientific research has determined that bodily movements are regulated by an area of the brain called the basal ganglia, whose cells require a proper balance of substances known as *dopamine* and *acetylcholine*, both involved in the transmission of nerve impulses. With Parkinson's, cells that produce dopamine begin to degenerate. When this happens, the insufficient dopamine disturbs the balance between dopamine and other transmitters, such as acetylcholine.

Therefore, dopamine can be seen as a chemical messenger responsible for transmitting signals between the substantia nigra and the next 'relay station' of the brain, which is the corpus striatum, to produce smooth, purposeful muscle activity. Loss of dopamine causes the nerve cells of the striatum to fire out of control, leaving the person unable to direct or control their movements in a normal manner.

The exact cause of this cell death or impairment is unknown. However, scientists have made advances in this area and one theory holds that free radicals, unstable and potentially damaging molecules generated by normal chemical reactions in the body, may contribute to nerve cell death that leads to Parkinson's.

Free Radicals and Anti-Oxidants

Free radicals are the highly unstable chemicals that attack, infiltrate and injure vital cell structures. Most stable chemical compounds in the body possess a pair of electrons. Sometimes, one member of the electron pair gets stripped away. The resulting compound (less one electron) is called a free radical.

The term 'free radical' means that it is now free to combine with another element to form a new stable compound. Free radicals can do a lot of damage by forming a chain reaction and breaking down other cell structures. A good comparison is that of the family unit. When two people join together and form a family unit, they are not usually available to other partners. However, if they separate the partners can go and look for another mate. Potentially, they can break up another stable marriage. This is the way free radicals work. When a free radical is born, it goes around the body looking for another compound to steal an electron from. While on the prowl, these free radicals can do tremendous damage to cells.

The most observed free radical chain reaction in living things is lipid peroxidation. The term lipid refers to any fat-soluble substance, animal or vegetable. Peroxidation means the formation of a peroxide molecule. These are the molecules with the greatest proportion of oxygen molecules.

Ninety-eight percent of the oxygen we breathe is used by tiny powerhouses within our cells called mitochondria, that convert sugar, fats and inorganic phosphate oxygen into adenosine triphosphate the universal form of energy that we need to live. This energy producing activity of the mitochondria involves a series of intricate complex and vital biochemical processes dependent on vast numbers of enzymes. These in turn are dependent upon dozens of nutrient factors and co-factors. In this metabolism process a very small amount of left over oxygen loses electrons, creating free radicals. These free radicals burn holes in our cellular membranes. Calcium penetrates our cells through these holes. This excess calcium results in cell death. This in turn weakens tissues and organs with the body, in turn weakening our overall immunity and resistance.

In addition to the oxygen that we breathe, the free radicals can also come from such things as environmental pollution, radiation, cigarette smoke, chemicals and herbicides.

Fundamental to having a healthy body is repairing the damage caused by the free radicals before it is too late and to protect the body's tissue cells from the free radicals before they cause mutations.

Antioxidants

Antioxidants are substances that have free radical chain reaction breaking properties. The antioxidants deactivate potentially dangerous free radicals before they can damage cells machinery. Most of these antioxidants come from plants and are called Phytochemicals. Among the most effective are vitamin A, C and E (known as the ACE trio against cancer). Out of these, vitamin C is the most effective. Each cell produces its own antioxidants. However, the ability to produce them decreases with age. That is why (see the chapter on diet) a diet rich in antioxidant and phytochemical rich fruits and vegetables supplemented with additional vitamins and minerals is important.

Genetics

Researchers think, as do a lot of doctor's, that Parkinson's has a genetic link. The genetic material that makes us who and what we are is stored in our chromosomes. Chromosomes consist of deoxyribonucleic acid (DNA) which in turn consists of genes, which are the blueprints for our inherited traits such as the colour of our eyes, height and numerous other characteristics and conditions such as cancers and diabetes. A number of studies have taken place to try to determine the genetic link but most have been inconclusive.

When assessing whether a disease is inherited, researchers will examine family history. It appears that the genetic link is strongest with first-degree relatives, i.e. parents, siblings and children. The larger the number of relatives with a specific condition the greater the likelihood that a genetic factor has played a direct role in transmission.

When it comes to Parkinson's, however, it seems that the jury is out and that there are differing opinions as to the importance of the genetic link. Some families have a clear pattern of Parkinson's disease within the family tree. Multiple family members across the generations have the condition. A study of a family, the Contursi family, revealed that 60 family members had Parkinson's disease over five generations. Autopsies of several family members showed the classic loss of dopamine cells and the presence of Lewy bodies.

Parkinson's disease and inheritance factors

The chart overleaf, compiled by Dr Jill Marjama-Lyons clearly demonstrates the risks of inheriting Parkinson's disease based on family history.

Person with Parkinson's disease in your family	Chance of getting Parkinson's disease
None	1-2 per cent, same as the general population
Brother or sister	5-6 per cent
One parent	10 per cent
Parent and sibling	20-40 per cent

As the table demonstrates, even if some family members have Parkinson's disease, there is no reason to assume that other family members will develop it as well. The risk may increase but there is nothing concrete by way of research to prove that this is absolutely the case.

Young-onset Parkinson's disease

Parkinson's disease is not solely a disease of the elderly. While the majority of cases are diagnosed in older people, it is estimated that about 15 per cent of people with Parkinson's disease develop symptoms before the age of 50. It has been established that the rate of young-onset Parkinson's disease is on the rise. Those who develop the disease prior to 55 years of age are considered to have young-onset Parkinson's disease. Very rarely, people under 21 will develop the disease, which is then classified as juvenile-onset Parkinson's disease.

Other factors

Research has been carried out on the influence of the environment as a factor in contributing to Parkinson's disease. There is no clear evidence to suggest that environment is major factor. Relatively weak influences have shown to be a possible factor, such as drinking water from a well, the proximity to wood mills, and the associated chemicals employed in these mills and also exposure to herbicides and pesticides, particularly among agricultural workers. However, such factors only contribute to a very small minority of cases.

Exposure to heavy metals, occupational exposure, such as copper, lead, iron, manganese and so on, increases the risk of developing Parkinson's by up to 10 times compared to the normal population. In addition, the iron and aluminium content is much higher than normal in the brains of people with Parkinson's disease.

Viral infections may also play a role in triggering Parkinson's disease. For example, during the outbreak of sleeping sickness during the First World War, about 15 million people were infected with the virus, and about 6 million of those developed Parkinson's symptoms. However, it was found later, during autopsies of some of the victims that the symptoms, although similar, weren't in fact Parkinson's.

Low levels of Estrogen

Some researchers believe that the female hormone estrogen may help protect against developing Parkinson's disease. This connection was supported by research published in the American journal *Movement Disorders* which compared the medical records of 72 women with Parkinson's disease and a group of women the same age who did not have the disease. The researchers found that the women who developed Parkinson's had three times the rate of hysterectomies, a higher rate of early menopause, and a lower rate of estrogen replacement therapy after menopause. The study suggested that estrogen may help to prevent or delay the onset of Parkinson's disease.

Caffeine and Nicotine

Caffeine has been blamed for many negative health effects. However, it has also been associated with a lower rate of Parkinson's disease. Numerous studies have shown that those who drink several cups of coffee a day have a lesser chance of developing Parkinson's disease than those who don't drink coffee. In addition, although cigarette smoking is very definitely harmful to health, ironically, people who smoke seem to have lower rates of Parkinson's disease than those who smoke. For reasons that are not clearly understood, nicotine appears to protect the dopamine producing cells in the brain.

This doesn't mean that you should take up smoking, far from it. Like a lot of studies, although the link between smoking and not developing Parkinson's was tenuously established, the fact is that smoking is a killer generally. So, if you don't smoke, don't start.

Diet and Nutrition

The exact relationship between diet and nutrition remains, like the other relationships, vague and controversial. Nothing that a person can eat, or not eat, has been definitely linked to Parkinson's. However, some researchers have shown that diet may help to prevent some cases of the disease. We will be discussing diet later on in the book, but briefly diets rich in antioxidants-such as vitamin C, Vitamin E and Beta-carotene-may help to reduce the levels of free radicals in the body, reducing the risk of developing Parkinson's disease.

Age related factors

In some individuals, the normal age-related wearing away of dopamine producing cells, plus the fact that we are living longer, accelerates the onset of Parkinson's disease. The older you get, whether male or female, the greater the chances of developing Parkinson's disease. The incidence of Parkinson's disease in the under 50's is less than 10 per 100,000 per year compared to more than 200 per 100,000 for those over 80. Parkinson's UK www.parkinsons.org.uk is in the process of funding many different research groups who are investigating all of the above areas in order to reach new conclusions in the causes and effects of Parkinson's.

In this chapter we have outlined the underlying causes of Parkinson's and also the potential contributory factors. As can be seen, there are a number of factors, however, research hasn't been conclusive and is still carrying on. Age and environmental influences seem to play a major role. In chapter two we will be looking at the diagnosis of Parkinson's disease and the importance of symptoms in recognising Parkinson's.

****

Chapter 2

The Diagnosis of Parkinson's Disease

As my own experience reflects, the diagnosis of Parkinson's disease has to be carried out very carefully and with certainty, as the consequences of a wrong diagnosis can be very stressful and traumatic for the person involved. In my case, once people, including in the first instance, my doctor, had convinced me that I had Parkinson's disease, I began to prepare myself for a life spent coping with the condition. It is therefore best not to listen to people around you, as everyone seems to be an amateur doctor, but make sure that you have specialist advice.

The main characteristics of Parkinson's disease
Although there are numerous symptoms of Parkinson's disease the main characteristics include slowness, general stiffness and an ongoing tremor.

Tremor
Tremor, which is the most common symptom associated with Parkinson's disease, is another term for shaking or trembling of the body. There are several types of tremor:

- Rest tremor, which occurs when the limb, usually wrist, fingers or arm, is relaxed and not in use. It ceases when the limb is in use.

- Postural tremor, which occurs when an arm or leg is held out against gravity, such as when holding a newspaper or book.
- Action tremor, as the name suggest this occurs when the limb is in use, such as when preparing food or eating.
- Pill rolling tremor, which occurs when rolling the thumb against the index finger.

Rigidity

Rigidity is a tightening or stiffening of the muscles. There are two basic types of rigidity, lead –pipe rigidity (the body won't move and is stiff, like a lead-pipe) and cogwheel rigidity (the body moves in a jerky motion, similar to the cogs in a wheel). In both types of rigidity the body does not move smoothly and there can also be pain.

The incidence of rigidity and overall stiffness will vary with individuals. Typically, rigidity occurs more on one side than the other and involves arms, legs, neck and back.

Bradykinesia

Bradykinesia is a general term referring to slowness of movement or speech. The term akinesia refers to absence of movement, which can also be a sign of Parkinson's disease. In most cases, akinesia shows up as an arm that does not swing when you walk or similar inability to move voluntarily.

Most people with Parkinson's disease experience some kind of bradykinesia, which can be experienced in a number of ways-from freeze attacks to difficulty dressing and walking to difficulty swallowing. These symptoms will come and go but when they are active the person may feel weakness.

Balance

Another very common symptom of Parkinson's disease is postural instability or problems with balance. Whilst this is not considered to be one of the major symptoms, many people with Parkinson's do have problems with their balance.

There are a number of other symptoms associated with Parkinson's such as light-headedness or fainting, problems with vision, problems with walking, weight loss, sleep problems and urinary problems. This list isn't exhaustive but your doctor, when assessing you for Parkinson's, or initially assessing your condition to determine whether or not it is Parkinson's will take them all into account.

The process of elimination

There is no specific diagnostic procedure or laboratory test to establish the diagnosis of Parkinson's disease. Therefore, a diagnosis is based on patterns. As the disease develops gradually, it is hard to be sure of a diagnosis until enough symptoms are present. Diagnosis is especially difficult in older people, because aging can cause some of the same problems as Parkinson's disease, such as loss of balance, slow movements, muscle stiffness and stooped posture.

Although there are no specific tests for Parkinson's disease, certain types of scans can provide evidence to support clinical diagnosis by measuring the ability of the brain to produce dopamine. These scans use processes called Positron Emission Tomography (PET) or Single Photon Emission Tomography (SPECT). These scans, however, are not used as a standard diagnostic test for Parkinson's disease. In my own case, I underwent a deep brain scan, which was an unpleasant experience, and it was this scan which provided conclusive evidence that my condition wasn't Parkinson's.

Carrying out the diagnosis

Given the difficult task of initially detecting Parkinson's disease, doctors usually have to carry out detective work, which is, essentially, a three-step process.

1. Assessing the symptoms

To diagnose Parkinson's disease, a doctor-preferably a neurologist or specialist-must carry out a review of the patients detailed medical history and perform a complete physical examination. The doctor will consider all the Parkinson's symptoms. In many cases, doctors will not consider Parkinson's as a possibility if there is not a tremor. However, as one in three people do not have tremors this is not really a very good starting point.

2. Consider all the possible diagnosis

After a detailed study of your symptoms, your doctor will need to look at the possibility of other diseases aside from Parkinson's. In the early stages, it can be very difficult to distinguish. Is arthritis present? Do you have a benign tremor? What exactly is happening? To make this determination, doctors should consider the fact that you may have another condition with symptoms similar to Parkinson's. There are a number of other possibilities:

Aging-this is the most obvious one. People tend to slow down as they get older. They walk more deliberately and experience problems with balance and also develop tremors, similar to Parkinson's.

Arthritis-this is another condition which has similarities to Parkinson's. Arthritis involves bone and joint pain, causing inflammation and loss of coordination. However, the symptoms of arthritis differ from Parkinson's in several ways:

- Arthritis is much easier to confirm with blood tests and x-rays.
- Arthritis causes joint pain and not muscle pain, as with Parkinson's
- Parkinson's symptoms don't respond to medication given for arthritis
- Arthritis doesn't cause tremors with muscle tone remaining normal.

Depression-depression can cause slow movement, stooped posture, weight loss and other common symptoms of Parkinson's. In addition, depression coexists alongside Parkinson's, making diagnosis more difficult. We will be discussing depression a little later in the book.

Essential tremor-many people, including medical people, confuse essential tremor with Parkinson tremor. Essential tremor is far more common than Parkinson's disease. People with essential tremor do not exhibit any other symptoms of Parkinson's disease, such as rigidity or problems with balance. Essential tremor is usually an action tremor that occurs on both sides, left and right while Parkinson's tremor usually appears at rest and only on one side.

Stroke-in some cases people with Parkinson's disease are diagnosed as having suffered a stroke because they present symptoms on one side of the body (this is most common when the person does not experience a tremor). In strokes, symptoms appear very quickly, whereas with Parkinson's they are gradual.

If, after exhaustive tests, Parkinson's is diagnosed, then a course of medication is prescribed to begin to try to establish a balance and rectify the perceived problems. Even at this stage, there is still a lot of uncertainty as Parkinson's disease is notoriously difficult to diagnose. It is only through time, and the onset of the condition, and trials with medication that the condition can be stabilized.

The next chapter deals with medication and the importance of getting the right medication, and also your role in identifying symptoms which in turn helps the doctor develop a successful program for you. Again, this chapter is not exhaustive as only a specialist can arrive at a correct dosage of the appropriate medication.

****

Chapter 3

Medication and Parkinson's

Having been through the initial, often traumatic, stages of the initial diagnosis, it is very necessary for you to build up a detailed knowledge of the type of medication that you will have to take for Parkinson's disease and also the side effects of that medication plus the effects of mixing medication.

In the first instance, if a doctor thinks that Parkinson's disease may be present, then, typically, a trial dose of dopamine-stimulating medication is administered. If, after this initial medication the patients condition improves then he or she is considered to have Parkinson's. If the patient does not improve then the doctor must consider another diagnosis.

Medications

Drugs that are currently in use to treat Parkinson's disease make movement easier and can prolong functions for many years. Overall, medications in use aim to replace, or to mimic, the missing chemical dopamine in the brain. The pharmacological treatment of Parkinson's is quite complex. While, overall, there are a large number of drugs that can be effective, their effectiveness will vary with the patient, the progression of the disease and the length of time that the medication has been used. Related side effects can preclude the use of certain medications, or require the introduction of a new drug to counteract them. Currently, there are five classes of drugs used to treat Parkinson's disease.

Drugs that replace dopamine

One particular drug that helps to replace dopamine is Levodopa (L-dopa) and is the single most effective treatment for the symptoms of Parkinson's disease. L-dopa is a derivative of dopamine, and is converted into dopamine by the brain. Doctors may choose to commence it when symptoms begin, or when they become serious enough to interfere with work or daily living.

L-dopa therapy usually remains effective for five years or longer. Following this, many patients develop motor fluctuations, including what is known as peak-dose dyskinesias (abnormal movements such as tics, twisting or restlessness) rapid loss of response after dosing and unpredictable drug response. Higher doses are usually tried, but may lead to an increase in dyskinesias. In addition, side effects of L-dopa may be nausea and vomiting, plus low blood pressure which can cause dizziness. These effects usually lessen after several weeks of therapy.

Enzyme inhibitors

Dopamine is broken down by several enzyme systems in the brain and elsewhere in the body and blocking these enzymes is a key strategy to prolonging the effect of a dose of dopamine. The two most commonly prescribed forms of L-dopa contain a drug to limit the amino acid and decarboxylase (an ADC inhibitor), one type of enzyme that breaks down dopamine. These combination drugs are Sinemet and Madopar. Controlled release formulations also aid in prolonging the effective interval of an L-dopa dose. The enzyme

Moncamine oxidase B (MAO-B) inhibitor selegiline may be given as an add-on therapy for L-Dopa. Research indicates that selegiline may have a neuroprotective effect, sparing nigral cells from damage by free radicals. Because of this, and the fact that it has few side effects, it is also frequently prescribed early on in the disease before L-Dopa is begun.

Dopamine agonists

Dopamine works by stimulating receptors on the surface of corpus striatum cells. Drugs which also stimulate these receptors are called dopamine agonists. Dopamine agonists are used both as adjuncts to levodopa therapy, and also initially in early Parkinson's disease, especially in young adults. The side effects of dopamine agonists are similar to those of levdopa, although they are less likely to cause involuntary movements and more likely to cause hallucinations or sleepiness.

This class of drugs includes the older dopamine agonists bromocripline (Partodel) and pergolide (permax) and the newer drugs pramipexole (Mirapex) and ropinirole (Requip). You should avoid dopamine agonists if you already experience hallucinations or confusion.

Anticholinergic drugs

Anticholinergics help control tremors in the early stages of the disease. Even so, they are only mildly beneficial and sometimes the benefits are offset by side effects such as dry mouth, nausea, urine retention, especially in men with enlarged prostrate-and severe constipation. These drugs can also cause or exacerbate mental problems, including memory loss, confusion and hallucinations.

Amantadine

Amantadine (Symadine, Symmeterel) stimulates the release of dopamine and may be used for patients with early mild symptoms. It has some benefit against muscle rigidity and slowness and may help older patients who are unresponsive to other drugs. It is less powerful than levodopa and may lose its effectiveness after about six months. It may also reduce motor fluctuations brought on by levadopa.

Using medications safely

There are basic guidelines for safe use of medication, listed below.

- Always continue with your course of medication and don't stop taking it unless you have consulted with your doctor. Appendix one shows an example of a medication log which should always be maintained so that you can produce evidence to your doctor if the medication is, in your opinion, not having the desired effect.

- Always begin medication with the lowest possible dose and increase gradually.

- If you experience side effects from Levdopa treatment ask your doctor about lowering the dose of the drug and adding a dopamine agonist.

- When changing a medication allow two to four weeks for your body to adjust before deciding that it is having a beneficial effect. It can take several weeks for your system to adjust to the new medication or dosage.

- Stick to a regular medication schedule, most important as keeping a steady amount of medication in your system will help reduce the likelihood of motor fluctuations.

- Before you take any new medication, ask your doctor to review the existing medications that you are taking and make sure that there are no side effects from mixing drugs.

The approach to treatment, and the administering of medications, differs for younger and older people. As a general rule, people over the age of 70 tend to take levdopa. Older people have trouble tolerating dopamine agonists without suffering side-effects, including confusion and hallucinations. Younger people often use dopamine agonists to manage their symptoms early in the disease, in part because younger people experience fewer side effects from these drugs than older people. In addition, younger people often have more time ahead of them to manage Parkinson's symptoms, and many of the drugs will eventually lose their effectiveness.

Whatever the combination of medication used, stay in control, make sure that you medicate regularly and always request information about drugs that you are using, particularly combinations of drugs.

In the next chapter, we will look at current surgery for Parkinson's disease and also at the ongoing research.

****

Chapter 4

Surgery for Parkinson's and Ongoing Research

Surgery for Parkinson's Disease

Over the years, surgery for Parkinson's has developed and improved, particularly so since the 1980's. While medication remains the first line of treatment, there are surgical options available which should also be considered. Deep Brain Stimulation is the more common form of surgery used on people with Parkinson's along with what is know as 'lesioning'.

Deep Brain Stimulation

In the late 1990's, deep brain stimulation revolutionized the surgical treatment of Parkinson's disease. The surgery involves inserting a thin wire and electrodes into the brain, linking the wire to a remote battery, and stimulating the brain at a high frequency. The electrodes are positioned in the brain; the wires run under the skin along the skull and down the neck, eventually crossing over to a pacemaker battery pack in the chest wall.

Deep Brain Stimulation does not reverse all the symptoms, but tends to improve symptoms to a level where they were several years before. The physical changes associated with DBS are determined by the positioning of the electrodes.

Lesioning-Pallidotomy and Thalamotomy

Lesioning involves using a heat sensitive probe to make a small hole in the brain that will alter motor function and relieve Parkinson's symptoms.

Pallidotomy

Pallidotomy is the most common lesioning surgery for Parkinson's disease and has been available for the last 50 years. This procedure can help relieve tremors, rigidity and bradykinesia (slowness of movement) by 15-20% and dyskinesia (abnormal movements other than tremor) by up to 80%. However, Pallidotomy doesn't help people with walking and balance. Pallidotomy is often recommended for people with Parkinson's symptoms that cannot be controlled with medication, as well as for those with disabling dyskinesia.

Thalamotomy

Thalamotomy can help reduce Parkinson's tremor and essential tremor by as much as 90% but does not significantly reduce rigidity or bradykinesia. For this reason, thalamotomy is typically used only on patients with tremor-predominant PD or severe essential tremor that does not respond to medication.

Cell implants

Research is under way to find a way to restore function to patients with Parkinson's disease by implanting cells into the damaged region of the brain. Cells from a patient's adrenal medulla (which normally produces neurotransmitter substances including dopamine) have been tried but little improvements in symptoms was found.

Mixed results have been obtained with cells taken from the brain of human foetuses. These cells develop into neurons of the type lost from the substantia nigra in Parkinson's disease. This is a very sensitive and intricate procedure and the results have been varied

Work is now taking place to develop human cells that can be grown in a laboratory and will produce dopamine, perhaps by altering the cells DNA. These cells may then be put into a special type of capsule that protects them but allows the dopamine to leave These capsules may be microscopic and suitable for inserting into the same area of the brain as foetal implants.

Stem cells from embryos

A further area of research is the use of stem cells from human embryos. These cells are at an immature, early stage of development and, with the correct genetic signal, can change into any type of cell, including nerve cells. This is what happens normally after fertilisation-the few cells that grow from the fertilised egg go on to develop into all the different types of cell that form a baby. Each cell in your body has the genetic information to become any type of cell, it just depends which genes are active. It is hoped that we can find out how to switch on the genes that convert stem cells into neurons for implantation to improve Parkinson's disease. This particular research is still at the early stage.

Growth factors

Growth factors are molecules that can be obtained from a variety of different cell types in the body. They occur naturally and are designed to encourage the growth and maturation of cells. Growth factors derived from the brain and glial cells (a type of cell in the brain) have both been used with success in animals and some Parkinson's disease patients. This research is still in the early stages but may become a useful treatment in the future.

Surgery is one option for people with Parkinson's disease. However, most people try to stabilise the condition with medication. This involves a relationship between you and your doctor. Establishing a strong relationship is of the utmost importance. This relationship must be characterized by trust and openness and also the sharing of information.

In appendix one I have inserted a medication log, which is the main way of compiling ongoing evidence which will inform the doctor and enable him or her to provide the best course of medication. The next chapter deals with your relationship with your doctor and also any specialists that you may see.

****

Chapter 5

Finding the Right GP/Consultant

It is a fact that many of us will place ourselves in the hands of our doctor's, or consultants, and implicitly trust them to look after us and give us the best advice possible. I am afraid that this is not always borne out by experience. The type of care and advice that you might receive very much depends on the attitudes of individual doctors, some of whom are better than others.

Whether you are in the process of confirming a diagnosis of Parkinson's or need to work with your doctor to manage your ongoing condition, it is absolutely essential that you choose a doctor that you feel comfortable with and that you trust. Normally, within a family doctor practice there are different doctors who tend to specialise. You must ensure that you find the doctor best suited to you. If you have any questions about your diagnosis be sure to seek a second opinion-don't just rely on the diagnosis and 'grin and bear' it. Don't feel afraid to change your doctor if you need to, it is your life and your well-being.

Right at the outset, you will want to identify a group of people who will support you through your condition. These will include:

- A general practitioner, i.e. your doctor, who will address your overall health care and needs and also provide referrals.

- From your doctor's recommendation, a neurologist, who will manage your Parkinson's disease
- A movement-disorders specialist if your neurologist doesn't have experience in this field. The neurologist will usually recommend such a person
- A physical therapist who will help you to develop an exercise regime suited to you
- A dietitian who will assist you with your diet.

It will be up to you to be proactive when establishing this group-you should take the initiative don't leave this to the professionals. My own experience has been that unless you ask you won't always get!

Of most importance, you will want people who have the most experience in treating people with Parkinson's disorders. This is essential. Never be afraid to ask questions about your condition, don't get sidetracked and make sure that you get the right answers. This is particularly the case with medication as, in the first throes of Parkinson's, medication can take some getting used to, with all sorts of side effects. It is this area that you will need to ensure that you get right.

These are a number of very important questions that you should ask a doctor:

1. Can you determine the reason I developed Parkinson's disease?
2. Do you have experience of working with Parkinson's patients?
3. How many patients do you see on a regular basis?

4. What are my treatment options?

5. What are the pros and cons of each treatment?

6. What short-term and long-term side effects can I anticipate from the treatment? Is there anything I can do to minimise them?

7. Can you recommend any support groups for my family and me?

8. Are there any non- medication options that might help? What lifestyle modifications can I make to help me feel better?

9. Are there any foods, supplements or over-the-counter medications I should avoid?

10. Where can I find more information about the illness?

11. Can you recommend any relaxation and stress-relief techniques?

12. Are there any clinical trials I can participate in?

13. What is your personal opinion about surgery for Parkinson's?

14. What is the success rate using surgery?

15. What is your opinion about alternative therapies?

16. Who will cover for you if you are away and I have problems?

Ultimately, as with any condition, it is vitally important that you communicate with your GP and take the lead. This will ensure that you get the best possible treatment.

One final tip is to always, if possible, try to maintain a record of your symptoms. See the appendix for a sample log. This will ensure that you can demonstrate clearly to the doctor what exactly the problems are and how frequently they occur.

Always keep a record of the medications that you are using and bring this to the doctors with you. Whilst it is true that the doctor will also have records it is important that you are in control as well as the doctor.

If you feel that it is necessary you should also bring a friend or carer to the doctors appointment with you as they can provide clarification and support. When you are with the doctor, you should not wait for the doctor to ask you about your most pressing concerns but you should outline these concerns right at the outset. Although doctor's are qualified they don't know everything and the dialogue between you and your doctor is a two-way process. Tell the doctor everything, even the most embarrassing symptoms that you would rather keep to yourself. It is very important to ensure that he or she has a clear picture of what is happening.

In the next chapter, we will look at the onset of depression and how it affects people with Parkinson's and how to combat it. I have also outlined a number of groups which play an important role in supporting people with Parkinson's.

****

Chapter 6
Combating Depression

Parkinson's and depression

When a person is diagnosed with Parkinson's, the trauma of that diagnosis can easily lead to depression. It is also common for depression to stay with a person, on and off, for many years. As depression can be debilitating, it is very important that you learn to recognise it and handle it to minimise the impact.

Factors contributing to depression

Living with Parkinson's means living with a situation where you are no longer functioning as you were. It is difficult to do the things that you once did and the knowledge that the condition is degenerative also has a negative impact. In addition, your brain chemistry has altered causing biochemical depression.

There are certain warning signs indicating clinical depression, as distinct to the common form of sadness felt by many Parkinson's sufferers.

- Changes in sleep patterns can be an early warning sign
- Changes in weight or eating habits
- Chronic fatigue or ongoing tiredness
- Apathy-although this is often a by-product of Parkinson's and can be distinct from depression
- Inability to concentrate or think clearly
- Withdrawal or isolation

- Anger and irritability
- Frequent crying
- Thoughts of suicide
- Apprehension about the future.

For most people with Parkinson's, depression is an organic illness involving both physical and biochemical changes in the body. It is very important to get the right medication at the early stages to minimise these changes. It is also crucial to ensure that you have access to counselling and professional care.

When it comes to treating depression, most mental health professionals rely on three specific forms of treatment, counselling or talking cures, medication (drug therapy) and, in the most extreme cases, ECT or Electro-Convulsive therapy. Usually, a combination of counselling and medication is used in the first instance and has the greatest success rate.

In most cases, depression usually responds relatively quickly to medication, such as drugs that inhibit the reuptake of seretonin (SSRI's) allowing the seretonin in the body to work longer. If you are in medication for depression you need to allow time for the drugs to work. Anti-depressants often take several weeks to lift the symptoms of depression. Medication should be used for several months during an initial period. You should work with your doctor to explore a range of treatments, until you find one suitable for you.

The importance of working towards acceptance of Parkinson's

When people are first diagnosed with Parkinson's, they almost always go through a process of grieving. It is essential that, during this period, you allow yourself to ride the emotional roller coaster associated with grieving. The five stages of grieving that have been identified are:

- Denial and isolation
- Anger
- Bargaining
- Depression
- Acceptance

Acceptance is the stage that you want to arrive at but you won't get there unless you have travelled through the other stages. The ongoing challenge with Parkinson's disease is that, once you have reached the stage of acceptance, you experience another setback or new symptoms that may require you to start the process over again. However, once you have reached the stage of acceptance then you will almost certainly be resilient enough to carry on.

It is very difficult indeed, in practice, to remain stoic when you are experiencing the ongoing conditions associated with Parkinson's. It is also very difficult for partners or those around you. The most important element here is having a knowledge of the condition and a future, forward looking philosophy that will take you through the dark times and allow you to focus on the future.

The importance of support groups

In the light of what we have just discussed, and the fact that most peoples personal circumstances differ, some have family, children and grandchildren, parents and so on, some people have no one, it is very important that people with Parkinson's have access to support groups. Within support groups you can share experiences and begin to understand that you are not alone with the condition. You can form new friendships and also gain invaluable advice about day-to-day living.

You will find many useful addresses at the rear of the book which can point you in the right direction, particularly in your own area. One of the first ports of call is Parkinson's UK, formerly the Parkinson's Disease Society, address and website below and at the back of the book. This organisation provides a wealth of information and advice and guidance about Parkinson's disease. Below are some of the groups in alphabetical order and which are repeated in the back of the book.

European Parkinson's Disease Association (EPDA)

1 Cobden Road
Sevenoaks
Kent
TN13 3UB
United Kingdom
e-mail: info@epda.eu.com

Umbrella body for network of international Parkinson's disease groups, campaigning on behalf Of all suffers. Information leaflets on request. An S.A.E. requested. EPDA has reports of all current research carried out to date, such as medication and surgical advances and also publishes a magazine called Parkinson's Life.

Leonard Cheshire Disability
66 South Lambeth Road
London
SW8 1RL
Tel: 020 3242 0200
www.lcdisability.org
Email: info@lcdisability.org
Contact Customer Helpline on 0808 808 2236 email
customerhelpline@lcdisability.org

National offices
Leonard Cheshire Disability Scotland
Murrayburgh House
17 Corstorphine Road
Edinburgh
EH12 6DD
Tel: 0131 346 9040
Fax: 0131 346 9050
email: scotlandoffice@LCDisability.org

Leonard Cheshire Disability Wales
Leonard Cheshire Disability Wales
Llanhennock Lodge
Llanhennock
Nr Caerleon
NP18 1LT
Tel: 01633 422583
Email: walesoffice@leonardcheshire.org

Leonard Cheshire Disability Northern Ireland
5 Boucher Plaza
4-6 Boucher Road
Belfast
BT12 6HR
Tel: 028 9024 6247
Fax: 028 9024 6395
email: northernirelandoffice@LCDisability.org

Leonard Cheshire Disability offers care, support and a wide range of Information for disabled people aged between 18 and 65 years in the UK and worldwide to encourage independent living. Has respite and residential homes; offers holidays and rehabilitation.

Parkinson's UK
National Office
215 Vauxhall Bridge Road
London
Hepline: 0808 800 0303
Tel: 020 7931 8080
Fax: 020 7233 9908
www.parkinsons.org.uk
Email: hello@parkinsons.org.uk

Northern Ireland office
Parkinson's UK Northern Ireland
Wellington Park Business Centre
3 Wellington Park
Malone Road
Belfast BT9 6DJ

Phone: 028 9092 3370
Email: northernireland@parkinsons.org.uk

Scotland office
Parkinson's UK Scotland
Suite 1-14
King James VI Business Centre
Riverview Business Park
Friarton Road
Perth
PH2 8DY
Phone: 0344 225 3724
Email: scotland@parkinsons.org.uk

Wales office
Parkinson's UK Wales/Cymru
Maritime Offices
Woodland Terrace
Maesycoed
Pontypridd CF37 1DZ
Phone: 0844 225 3784
Email: wales@parkinsons.org.uk

Offers information and support via its local groups Has nurse specialists and welfare department, And funds research into Parkinson's disease.

Patients' Association
PO Box 935
Harrow

Middlesex

HA1 3YJ

Helpline: 0845 608 4455

Tel: 0208 423 8999

www.patients-association.com

Email: helpline@patients-association.com

Provides advice on patients' rights, leaflets and also a directory of self-help groups.

Disability Rights UK

Ground Floor

CAN Mezzanine

49-51 East Rd

London

N1 6AH

www.disabilityrightsuk

Tel: 0207 250 8181

Campaigns to improve the rights and care of Disabled people. Sells special key to access locked disabled toilets.

Revitalise (previously Vitalise)

212 Business Design Centre

52 Upper street

London N1 OQH

General enquiries 0303 303 0145

www.vitalise.org.uk

Offers holidays at their own centres and overseas and respite care for people with severe disabilities by Providing voluntary carers. Also arranges holidays for people with alzheimer's disease/dementia and their carers.

YPN (Younger Parkinson's Network)

National helpline : 0808 800 0303

The young-onset self-help group of the Parkinson's Disease Society is designed really for those of Working age. There are around 1,300 members of YPN , many of them in their early 20s and 30s. Has a magazine, local meetings and conference every 2 years.

Network of local groups bringing people with Parkinson's and their families together for support and help.

Parkinson's Home Care

Helping Hand Homecare

Arrow House

8-9 Church Street

Alcester

Warwickshire

B49 5AJ

0843 634 4883

www.helpinghandscare.co.uk

One of the most invaluable resources available to you is the internet. You can locate support groups local to you by surfing the web. In addition, Libraries are invaluable sources of information.

If you have, or you think that you have Parkinson's then there is a wealth of information out there to help you make contact with a variety of organisations that will be ready and able to assist you.

In the next chapter, we will move on to discussing the importance of diet and nutrition for those with Parkinson's. Many of the tips are universal and are common sense to all people. However, they are particularly important for those with Parkinson's.

****

Chapter 7

Diet and Parkinson's Disease

Whilst there is no special diet in use for people with Parkinson's disease, as with all people a well-balanced nutritious diet is an absolute must and will, in the long term, prove beneficial. It is a well known fact that with a proper diet, our bodies work more efficiently and we feel a lot more healthy. The upshot of this is that Parkinson's disease medications will work properly and more effectively with a well-balanced diet.

We (the authors) are not specialist dietitians and make no recommendations based on any specialism. The information contained below is based on good common sense and information gleaned from specialist publications.

Eating well with Parkinson's

Generally, Parkinson's patients should eat a well balanced diet, high in fruits and vegetables and relatively low in protein. The following represents sound guidelines for people with PD.

It is generally accepted that people with Parkinson's should eat more fibre. This helps to prevent constipation and helps to speed food through the digestive tract, minimising the amount of time that food remains in the intestines. Most people eat about 15 grams of fibre daily. Those with Parkinson's should strive to eat about double that amount. A useful source of fibre is dried fruit. You should also switch from refined to whole grains. You may also want to consider fibre supplements. Add these supplements to your diet slowly to avoid side effects which can include gas or diarrhoea.

In addition, it helps if Parkinson's sufferers drink lots of water. This helps with constipation and also helps with the respiratory system, acts as a lubricant and flushes waste through the bloodstream. It is a fact that some Parkinson's medication can contribute to dehydration. A good daily intake of water is around eight 8-ounce glasses per day. This should, ideally, be filtered or bottled water.

It is also well worth considering probiotics, or yoghurt. The 'good' bacteria found in yoghurt with live cultures and supplements help complete the digestive process, reduce inflammation and balance the endocrine system. You can obtain such foods from good health food stores and also pharmacies.

Like a lot of people with any sort of condition, it is best to avoid spicy foods. Some people with Parkinson's find that they experience violent dyskinesia after they eat spicy foods. It is best to give such foods a miss.

It is a fact that people with Parkinson's can be susceptible to thinning bones caused by osteoporosis. Foods high in calcium, magnesium and vitamin D should be consumed, timed to complement your medication. The maintenance of a healthy weight is very important and you will need to watch your calorie intake so that you can maintain your ideal weight. Some people with Parkinson's will lose weight (tremors and dyskinesia can burn an excessive amount of calories) others will gain weight as a result of the side effects of some medications).

Underweight

You may find that you are underweight and have difficulty putting weight on. Sometimes, weight loss can be due to practical problems to do with food preparation and keeping your food hot while you are eating.

The way you buy, store, prepare and cook food may need a little rethinking. It is recommended that you seek advice from an occupational therapist who can advise you on all aspects of food shopping and preparation, including kitchen and shopping aids. Here are a few tips:

- You should always try to plan your meals in advance, making a shopping list of all the necessary ingredients.
- When you are planning meals, you should decide how long you should stand at a cooker before you get tired.
- You should consider buying foods that are already prepared, such as frozen foods like vegetables and tinned fish, meat or beans. Ready meals will save time on all fronts.
- Keep well stocked with a wide supply of food.
- If you can, purchase a microwave, as they will save a lot of time.
- If you like a nap in the afternoon, keep hot water in a flask on a tray with a tea bag, milk, sugar etc. Drinking regularly helps you to keep warm

- You may be entitled to meals on wheels or home delivery of frozen meals. You should contact the home care organiser of your local social services department.

Dishes and cutlery

There are a variety of adapted utensils for eating and drinking which may be worth buying. However, it is strongly recommended that you seek the advice of an occupational therapist before buying expensive specialised equipment.

Specialised cutlery is available in various shapes and sizes and you should use large mugs for drinks, but only half-full. Two-handled cups can improve grip and reduce the chance of spillage. Special 'tumble-not' mugs are available with wide, non-slip bases and tall necks.

A 'stay-warm' plate might be useful if it takes you a long time to eat, or you could have smaller, more frequent meals. A damp cloth placed under a plate will stop it from slipping, or special mats can be used. High lipped plates are available that prevent spillage and make it easier to draw food onto the fork or spoon. Similarly, plate guards can be bought that clip onto your usual plates. Equipment is also available to help with opening jars and bottles. Information on all of the above specialist equipment can be obtained from Parkinson's UK.

Advice on eating and swallowing food

As important as diet, and the preparation of food, is how you eat. The following tips might be helpful:

- Take your time when you eat. Eat in a comfortable, quiet setting. However, if you feel that you are taking too long and your food is getting cold, consider eating smaller more frequent meals, or food that is easier to eat.
- Try eating in the recommended eating position. This is sitting upright in a chair with both feet on the floor and the arm that you are not using resting on the table.
- Try planning your meals for when your medication is working. You should avoid eating large meals when you are off your medication.
- Some people feel their throats tense up while eating and food sticks in their throat. You should try yawning before a meal to relax your throat.

Some people find certain foods more difficult to chew or swallow than others. If this is the case then you may want to consider a semi-solid diet. However, before you do so, you should speak to a registered dietitian or your GP who can advise you. This is because not all swallowing problems are to do with Parkinson's and it is necessary to confirm the cause of the problem before changing diet. You can also be advised on the best consistency and texture of food/liquid for you.

Semi-solid foods are generally easier to swallow than foods with mixed textures or very hard or dry foods.

Tips on easier swallowing:

- Try slightly thicker creamy soups rather than watery ones, or those with 'bits' in.

- Meat that is tough or chewy can be difficult. Try moistening this with either gravy or some kind of sauce, or try fish, which is usually softer.
- Try mashed potato, pasta or noodles as a change from bread.
- Try wholemeal instead of white bread as white bread can get stuck in the mouth.
- Try soft, moist biscuits, such as sponge fingers rather than drier crackers or toast.
- Having a drink with your meal makes chewing softer. Iced water in particular may help the 'strength' of your swallow.
- Good posture and a comfortable position when eating will also aid swallowing.
- Try taking smaller mouthfuls.
- If you wear dentures make sure that they fit properly.

Puree diets

If you find swallowing very difficult, you should again seek advice from suitably qualified people, such as a GP, dietitian or therapist. They might suggest that you try a puree diet.

Below are some tips on a puree diet.

- If foods are being liquidised or pureed, always use a milk based sauce or gravy, rather than water. This will increase the nutrients and energy of the meal.
- Do not use baby foods; although they may be the right texture, they are not nutritionally adequate for adults.
- Thickening agents can be added to liquidised or pureed foods to add back some of the texture. Suitable thickeners

include milk powder, instant potato powder, custard powder or plain yoghurt.

Speech and language therapists, occupational therapists and registered dietitians can also advise further on diet, utensils and eating techniques. Again, there is plenty of information on the web site of Parkinson's UK related to diet.

A sample eating plan

As has been outlined above, and is also common sense, good nutrition in Parkinson's involves eating regularly, and also eating a wide range of different foods.

Overleaf is a sample eating plan with a variety of foods from which you can choose. Please bear in mind that this is only a sample and that you should pick and choose from what has been outlined.

See overleaf.

Breakfast	Fruit or fruit juice; cereal and milk; bread toast and butter (or margarine, soya spread etc) eggs, bacon, sausage etc; tea, coffee or milk.
Midday meal:	Meat, fish, eggs or cheese or alternative(consider cholesterol) Potato, rice, pasta or bread/toast;vegetables, yoghurt, custard or fruit drink.
Evening meal	Soup of fruit juice; meat, fish, eggs, beans or lentils, potato, rice, pasta, bread: salad or vegetables, yoghurt, ice cream and jelly
Between meals	Have a drink between meals, as well as with them, for example tea, coffee, soup, fruit juice, water etc. You can also snack lightly.
The main meals, midday and evening are interchangeable.	

Parkinson's medication and the interaction with food

Each of the medications in use with Parkinson's disease has a particular interaction with food. For example, levdopa generally works better when taken on an empty stomach. Therefore your doctor may possibly prescribe a combination of levdopa and carbidopa (known as sinemet) or carbidopa by itself (called

Lodosyn). If nausea is a continual problem, then another drug may be prescribed to relieve these symptoms.

Controlling nausea

Given that nausea can be a problem with Parkinson's patients, it is useful to understand the best ways to control nausea. The following are useful tips:

- Drink clear or ice cold drinks. Drinks containing a small amount of sugars may calm the stomach better than other liquids.
- Avoid acidic drinks such as orange or grapefruit juices as they may worsen nausea.
- Drink liquids in between meals instead of during them.
- Avoid fried, greasy foods (always best avoided in all circumstances).
- Eat slowly, don't bolt food and eat smaller more frequent portions instead of large meals.
- Don't mix hot and cold foods. Eat foods that are cold at room temperature.
- Rest after you eat, don't rush around as this will bring on nausea.

Vitamins and minerals

Eating a well-balanced diet will provide adequate levels of vitamins and minerals for most people. Food contains fibre and other valuable nutrients, as well as vitamins and minerals. Essentially, if you feel that you are in need of more of a particular vitamin or mineral, it is usually advised that you eat more of the particular food containing them rather than buying expensive supplements.

In the next chapter, we will look at the benefits of exercise and Parkinson's disease. Exercise compliments diet and the two can combine to make you a healthy and able to cope better with life and your condition.

****

Chapter 8

The Benefits of Exercise and Parkinson's

Most people with Parkinson's understand the importance of exercise in the control and improvement of the disease.

Research has shown that there are several types of muscle weakness involved with Parkinson's, including weakening of the pulmonary muscles. Although those with Parkinson's will find it difficult at times to carry out exercises, it is important that a regular regime is adhered to.

The benefits of exercise
Exercise offers significant health benefits for everyone, whether or not they have Parkinson's disease. Exercise improves emotional and physical health, reduces risk of serious illness and increases overall energy levels. For those with Parkinson's regular exercise can help improve flexibility, reduce muscle stiffness and slow the advancement of Parkinson's symptoms.

Putting together an exercise plan
A well-rounded exercise plan includes three main components: aerobic fitness, muscle strength and flexibility.

Aerobic fitness
The word *Aerobic'* means 'using oxygen'. During aerobic exercise, your heart and lungs work harder than normal to provide muscles

with the oxygen they demand, and you breath heavily and steadily to meet your body's increased need for oxygen. During an aerobic exercise, your heart and lungs cannot meet your body's increased need for oxygen for longer than a minute or two, and you are left gasping for breath, even if you are in fairly good condition. Simple aerobic exercises include jogging and running short distances.

Jogging and running may not be everyone's idea of fun and there are alternatives to this. Swimming is a very good exercise as are other forms of gym exercise. The important thing is to find an exercise that is suitable for your condition and temperament.

Numerous studies have found that aerobic exercise not only helps people with Parkinson's disease improve their aerobic capacity, but it also helps with movement problems, such as freezing.

When choosing an aerobic activity, you need to find an exercise that involves the rhythmic, repeated use of the major muscle groups, such as walking, yoga, or tai chi. When done regularly-for example three times a week for at least 20-30 minutes at a time-aerobic exercises improve the efficiency of the heart, lungs and muscles.

To derive the maximum benefit from these exercises, you need to work hard enough, but not too hard, particularly in the beginning and also if you need to lose some weight. You need to ease in slowly but surely. Your pulse rate (heart beats per minute) is your body's speedometer. It tells you how fast your heart is going and if you need to speed up or slow things down. Cardiovascular conditioning takes place when your heart beats at 70-85 per cent of its maximum safe rate. Your maximum heart rate is approximately 220 minus your age.

Dancing or exercising to music is seen as beneficial. Studies have found that people with Parkinson's disease who participated in music therapy-including rhythmic and free body movement-experienced significant reduction in bradykinesia (slowness of movement and rigidity). In addition to regular workouts, it is important that Parkinson's sufferers remain as active as possible at all times. This can involve any type of activity, such as shopping, walking around the garden or playing with children or grandchildren.

Improving muscle strength

Whilst Parkinson's sufferers are prone to muscle weakness and atrophy, they are not particularly side effects of Parkinson's or inevitable effects of aging. However, they do happen and there is only one way to combat this and that is through exercise. You can keep muscles strong and supple by performing strength- building exercises, such as weightlifting and isometric exercises.

Strength training also helps stabilize the joints and reduce risks of falling and injury. It has been proven that strength training also helps people with Parkinson's disease improve their walking velocity and stride length. Since most people with Parkinson's disease have some trouble with walking or gait at some time, it is clear that some type of strength training should be some part of your exercise programme. Without strength training, you will lose muscle mass and strength. The average person will lose 10-20 percent of muscle strength between the ages of 20 to 50, and then another 25 to 30%

between 50 to 70. However, this can be held at bay, or slowed, by strength training.

Flexibility

Flexibility is the opposite of rigidity, which is one of the defining characteristics of Parkinson's disease. Flexibility involves maintaining the range of motion in your joints, which can allow you to perform your everyday activities without discomfort. Maintaining flexibility makes you less prone to muscle strains and sprains, and helps you support your joints.

Stretching is the key to preserving your flexibility. Begin with 10-minute stretching sessions in the morning and evening and work your way towards 20-minute sessions twice a day. You should move and stretch your entire body-neck, shoulders, waist, fingers, wrists, elbows, arms, toes, ankles, legs and hips-through their full range of motion in every direction. You should gently stretch and hold, then repeat two or three times. Only stretch to levels that you are comfortable with, don't overstretch as this can make things worse.

Stretch your facial muscles by opening your jaw, raise eyebrows, smile make facial expressions. Try to massage your face gently to reach the tiny muscles in your face. You need to talk to your GP or a therapist about a full list of stretching exercises, as you should for all other exercises.

Starting your exercises

For some people, it might be better to get a partner to help them begin exercising. This can be for the pleasure of exercising with someone else and also for practical reasons, such as someone to help you with balance and to assist you if you fall over. A very good option is to join a local group at a community centre or clinic. This might motivate you to maintain continuity. You can also share experiences.

Never do more than you can manage and never do any exercise that causes pain. You don't want to pull muscles or irritate joints. Organisations such as Parkinson's UK can give guidance on various forms of exercise and offer recommended programmes of exercise.

The next chapter looks at rights in the workplace and what to do if you are diagnosed with Parkinson's whilst at work or are looking for a job after a diagnosis of Parkinson's. for people with Parkinson's

****

Chapter 9

Employment and Parkinson's

Employment and Parkinson's

If you have Parkinson's, or you care for someone who does, you may have concerns about your working life. Work is not only a way of making a living, it can also be important for confidence, self-esteem and personal satisfaction.

If your treatment is carefully managed and you have plenty of support, it is possible to continue working for many years, depending on the type of job you have and how Parkinson's affects you. Speak to your GP, specialist or Parkinson's nurse about treatments to help you manage your symptoms and stay in work. Sometimes, changes need to be made to make work easier, such as reducing your hours, changing career or taking early retirement.

If you are in paid work and care for someone with the condition, you may find that, as time goes on, combining your responsibilities can be challenging. You may also need to make changes to maintain your general health and well being.

The most important thing to do is stay as informed as you can about what your rights are in the work place and use all the support networks available to you.

Discrimination in the workplace

Because Parkinson's is a long-term condition you are likely to meet the statutory (legal) definition of disabled under the Equality Act 2010, or the Disability Discrimination Act 2006 in Northern Ireland.

This means that it is unlawful for an employer to discriminate against you because of your disability or because of something that happens as a consequence of your disability. Employers also have a duty to make changes to the way you work to help you continue doing your job. These are known as reasonable adjustments (see page 9).

These laws protect anyone who has a physical or mental impairment that has a long-term, substantial adverse effect on their normal day-to-day activities.

Looking for a job when you have Parkinson's

If you are looking for a job you may be wondering about how much you should tell a possible employer about your condition.

In Northern Ireland employers are still allowed to ask questions about health and disability before making a job offer and may ask you to complete a pre-employment health questionnaire. You should answer the questions on the form honestly.

But remember that the Equality Commission for Northern Ireland says that a response to a medical questionnaire, the results of a medical examination or the opinion of a Medical Advisor should only be one of a number of factors that an employer should consider in reaching their final decision about who to hire. In particular, your potential employer should also consider what reasonable adjustments, if any, may be required. They should then make their selection decision following an assessment of how you would perform in the job if these reasonable adjustments were made.

In Great Britain it is against the law for a potential employer to ask you about your health or any disability before offering you a job, except in very limited circumstances.

You should only be asked health-related questions when they're necessary for certain purposes, including the following.

- If a potential employer is trying to find out whether you need any changes or reasonable adjustments to be made to the recruitment process (for example, the time or place of the interview because of a disability or health condition).
- If you are applying as a disabled person under the government's 'Two Ticks' symbol or any similar schemes to improve employment rates for people with a disability. Note that the Two Ticks scheme is not applicable in Northern Ireland.
- For monitoring purposes. Potential employers can ask you to complete a form giving your race, gender, sexuality, religion, age and if you have a disability. Filling in these forms is usually optional and should not be part of your application.

- If a potential employer is trying to find out if you have a disability or health condition that would affect your ability to carry out an essential part of the job. For example, if you were applying for a job as a builder your employer could reasonably ask you if you have any condition that would affect your ability to climb scaffolding and work at heights.
- If they require an employee to have a particular disability or condition as part of the role they are recruiting for.

It is up to you whether you tell anyone about your condition. You only need to tell a potential employer about a disability if you think your Parkinson's may cause a health and safety risk either to you or to someone else. If you need your employer to make changes to the way you work, i.e. reasonable adjustments You may decide that you don't want to tell potential employers that you have Parkinson's. This may be because you don't feel comfortable telling people about your condition, you believe your symptoms won't interfere with your ability to do the job, you feel that, at this time, the fact that you have Parkinson's is irrelevant to your working life

On the other hand, you may decide you'd rather tell a potential employer about your condition. This may be because you prefer it when others know about your condition, your symptoms are quite noticeable and you want to explain these at your interview, you'd like to reassure your employer that you can do the job, perhaps with reasonable adjustments (if you think you need them)

If you do choose to mention your Parkinson's on your application or at interview, be prepared for the response. In Great Britain, an interviewer should accept what you have said and move on without asking you any further questions. This is because employers in Great Britain are not allowed to ask questions about health or disability before offering you a job.

In Northern Ireland potential employers are allowed to ask questions about your health, but they must be clear about what this information will be used for. For example, are they asking so they can consider what reasonable adjustments you may need?

Positive discrimination

Positive discrimination is when one person is chosen over another for a job because of their age, disability, marital status, race, sex or sexual orientation.

Generally, this is unlawful except in the case of disability. Both the Equality Act and the Disability Discrimination Act allow employers to actively seek people with a disability for a role in certain circumstances. The most common forms of positive discrimination are the following.

- The 'Two Ticks' or Disability Symbol. The Disability Symbol is awarded by Jobcentre Plus to employers who make a commitment to employ, keep and develop disabled employees. This includes a guarantee to interview a disabled person who can do the job. If you are looking for work you may want to look out for employers who display this symbol in their adverts. This scheme is not run in Northern Ireland but there may be others. See the nidirect website www.nidirect.gov.uk for details of positive discrimination schemes in Northern Ireland.

- Adverts for jobs that say that the employer wants someone with a particular type of disability. This is usually because the role is working with people with that disability, for example the Royal National Institute for the Blind might want to employ someone who has a visual impairment.

If you are working when you are diagnosed or living with Parkinson's, you may be wondering what you should tell your employer about your condition.

Telling a manager about your diagnosis

This is up to you, though there may be some factors that influence your decision. You don't have to tell your manager or anyone else at work about your Parkinson's unless:

- there is a health and safety risk (i.e. your condition means that either you or someone else may be at risk of harm)
- you need to change the way you work because of your symptoms. In this case you will need to ask your employer for a reasonable adjustment under the Equality Act or Disability Discrimination Act in Northern Ireland. Your employer will need to know how your disability makes it difficult for you to do your job.

Unless you work in a small organisation without a human resources function, your manager doesn't normally need to know that you have Parkinson's. You can just say that you have a health condition and you need to change the way you work (if this is the case).

Your manager will probably ask you to speak to someone in the human resources department and you may be referred to an occupational health specialist or other medical advisor. They will put a report together on how your condition affects your ability to do your job and what changes could be made to make sure you can keep working or remove any disadvantages you may have at work because of your disability.

If you work for a large organisation, they may have their own occupational health specialists. Smaller businesses may send you to a GP. The occupational health specialist or GP you're referred to will need to know your diagnosis and you should be asked to sign a consent form that lets them ask for reports from your own GP or specialist.

Remember that if you tell your manager about your condition, they must not tell anyone else without your consent, except in very limited circumstances. For example, they may have to tell human resources or other managers in order to comply with their legal obligations to you, such as their duty to look after your health and safety and to make reasonable adjustments under the Equality Act.

If they do tell anyone else about your condition outside of these circumstances, they may be breaking the law. This is because the Data Protection Act says that information about health is sensitive, personal data and may only usually be shared if you say so. If you do inform your manager and/or human resources department about your condition, you may find it helpful to ask for more information about their policies related to employees with a long-term condition.

Telling colleagues about your condition

It is entirely up to you whether you tell your colleagues about your condition. But the important thing to know is that you don't have to tell your colleagues if you don't want to.

Because you are under no obligation, you can take the time to decide what you think is best for you in terms of what, if anything, you tell your colleagues. You may want to think about things like how your condition may affect you and your colleagues in the workplace, how noticeable your symptoms are and what your relationship is like with the people you work with.

You may wish to discuss your decision with someone you trust outside of work or speak to others with similar experiences. If you do decide to tell your colleagues about your condition, you may like to spend some time thinking about what you want to tell them and how you want to do this. You may want to tell them about Parkinson's in detail or you may prefer to be less specific and just let them know you have a health condition.

You may find it helpful to talk to your manager about how to tell your workmates. For example, you can tell them yourself or ask your manager to do it for you.

What are reasonable adjustments?

If you have Parkinson's, you may have difficulties in relation to where you work.

These difficulties may put you at a substantial disadvantage compared to other employees without a disability. By law, your employer must help to overcome or lessen that disadvantage by making changes to parts of the premises or working arrangements. These changes are called 'reasonable adjustments'.

These may include the following.

- Making changes to the premises where you work (for example, steps or doors).
- Altering your job, which may involve giving some of your non-core work that is difficult for you to someone else, like the occasional need for travel or work at a different site.
- Moving you to another post or place of work (see page 16 for more on redeployment)
- A change in working hours
- Giving you training
- Giving you modified equipment, such as computer adaptations, large button telephones or adjustable chairs
- Making instructions and manuals easier to use
- Using a reader or interpreter
- Increasing supervision
- Providing an automatic car if you need to drive at work
- Arranging with a taxi firm to supply taxis that will be paid for by Access to Work

- Working from home for some or all of the time, with the right equipment.

This list doesn't cover everything, because what is reasonable and effective will be different for everyone. Alongside yourself, an occupational health advisor or an Access to Work assessor is best placed to identify what adjustments may help you.

Making a request for reasonable adjustments

If you are having problems doing your job or parts of your job, the first thing to do is talk to your manager. An employer is only obligated to make reasonable adjustments if they know, or could reasonably be expected to know, that you have a disability. So you do need to tell them that you have a disability, but remember that you don't have to tell them you have Parkinson's if you don't want to.

Try to explain what part of your job is causing a problem and what that problem is. For example, you may have difficulties travelling to work on public transport during rush hour because you can't get a seat and find it difficult to stand for long periods of time. Or you may have problems using equipment such as a keyboard or computer because of movement difficulties.

You may also have some suggestions for changes that will help you. These could be starting and finishing later in the day, or speech to text software installed on your computer. These may have been adjustments that worked for you in a previous job.

Don't worry if you don't have any suggestions for what reasonable adjustments may help you. Your manager should arrange for you to have an assessment with an occupational health adviser to find out what your problems are and to make suggestions for how they can be solved.

If your manager does not do anything to make the reasonable adjustments you need, you will need to contact the human resources department. You can also contact Access to Work and make an application for an assessment.

Take some time to think about what adjustments may help you, but remember that they have to be reasonable – i.e. something that your employer will be able to do.

If your employer is a member of the Business Disability Forum ask your manager to look at the website or call the advice line for practical advice on what to do, as well as information on what the law states. See the more information and support section for details of the Forum.

Workplace Adjustment Agreements

When you and your manager have agreed on some reasonable adjustments, it's a good idea to put them in writing. This is called a Tailored Adjustment Agreement or Workplace Adjustment Agreement.

The purpose of recording this agreement is to make sure that you and your employer have an accurate record of what has been agreed, reduce the need to rearrange your reasonable adjustments every time you change jobs, are relocated within the organisation or get a new manager and provide you and your line manager with a basis for discussion about your reasonable adjustments at any future meetings, such as your regular catch-ups or one to ones. (You should regularly review your adjustments with your manager to make sure they are still working and to agree and make any necessary changes)

You can download a template agreement from the Business Disability Forum address at the rear of this book.

Taking time off for medical appointments or treatments

You can ask to take time off work for your medical appointments or treatment as part of your reasonable adjustment agreement.

Talk to your manager about how much time you think you need. If the appointments are for fixed times and you know well in advance, your employer should be able to allow you to take the time off you need.

Sick leave

If you are too unwell to work you may need to take time off sick. Time off sick is unplanned. Under these circumstances you should follow your employer's usual procedure on reporting sickness.

This will include telling your employer immediately that you're not able to work. If you're off sick for more than seven days, you will need to arrange getting a doctor's 'fit note' to give to your employer. If you are off sick due to your Parkinson's symptoms and haven't told your employer about your condition yet, you may feel it's best to do so before they receive a fit note or letter from your doctor.

Returning to work

If you've taken some time off and your employer is aware of your disability, their policies may allow you to have a few days more for sick leave than other employees before they start attendance improvement procedures.

Some employers ask on their sickness certificate that you complete when you return to work if your absence was related to a disability. If you want your employer to know that you have a disability or if you think you need to change the way in which you work (i.e. reasonable adjustments), you should say yes to this question. This may mean that you have to see an occupational health adviser or other medical advisor who will ask you about your symptoms and the way they affect you at work.

If you've been on sick leave for more than a few days, your employer may ask you to see their occupational health adviser or other medical advisor before your sick pay entitlement has expired. If there is medical evidence that your Parkinson's means you are more likely to need more time off sick than other people, this is a good opportunity to agree on some reasonable adjustments to prevent you taking time of sick. For example, you may find it helps to work from home from time to time.

Access to Work programme

An Access to Work grant is money for practical support to people with a disability, such as a long-term health condition.

The Access to Work programme is administered by Jobcentre Plus or Jobs and Benefit Offices in Northern Ireland. It is there to provide help towards covering the costs of adjustments, which otherwise would not be reasonable (e.g. they would be too expensive for your employer). Your employer still has a duty to make reasonable adjustments under the Equality Act and the Disability discrimination Act.

Applications for Access to Work must be made by the person with the disability on the application form.

If you're in England, Scotland or Wales contact your regional Access to Work centre for more information or to apply. Contact details can be found at the back of the book. An adviser will then contact you and your line manager to arrange for an appraisal of your needs.

You can also visit www.gov.uk/access-to-work to find out more about the scheme.

If you're in Northern Ireland, you should contact an Employment Service Adviser in your local Jobs and Benefits office or JobCentre. You can find out where this is by calling the free phone number 0800 353 530.

You can also visit www.nidirect.gov.uk to find out more about the scheme.

Discrimination

This information applies whether you are a person with Parkinson's or if you care for someone with the condition.

If you feel you are being treated unfairly in the workplace, the first thing to do is talk to your line manager. Ask for a meeting and talk to them about what has been happening (for example, you may feel you are being discriminated against because the reasonable adjustments you requested haven't been made or you feel a colleague is treating you unfairly).

If your line manager is the problem, then you need to talk to their manager or the human resources manager. It's best to start with an informal discussion. Your employer may simply not realise what difficulties you may be having or be aware of their legal obligations. If you explain what you need they may be willing to make the necessary changes.

If you are uncomfortable about talking to your employer alone there are things you can do. If are a member of a union, you can ask a trade union representative to go with you or you can ask if you can bring a colleague of your choice with you to the meeting. You can also ask your employer to allow a family member or trusted friend to be there with you for moral support.

If, after the informal meeting, you are still unhappy, you should make a formal complaint or grievance. Your staff handbook should tell you the process for doing this, or you should ask for guidance from human resources department on the employer's policies.

You will also need to find out more about your legal rights. Your trade union, the Equality and Human Rights Commission (EHRC), the Citizens Advice Bureau or the Equality Commission for Northern Ireland should be able to provide you with advice. See the back of this book for more details.

Ending work

If you are dismissed because of your disability or because your employer doesn't want to make reasonable adjustments you may be able to make a claim for disability discrimination and/or unfair dismissal.

You must find out what rights you have to bring a claim and what you should do next as soon as possible because strict time limits apply to making claims to the employment tribunal.

If you have been given a warning about your performance or conduct at work, you may be at risk of dismissal and should seek advice immediately. This can be from your Trade Union if you are a member, your local Citizens Advice Bureau or Law Centre or from the Disability Law Service.

Redundancy

The information on redundancy applies whether you are a person with Parkinson's or if you care for someone with the condition.

If all the correct procedures are followed, redundancy is a lawful and fair way of dismissing employees that the employer no longer has work for. Your employer can only lawfully make you redundant if:

- the business as a whole is closing
- a particular branch, office or workplace is closing
- fewer employees are needed to do particular work
- the job you are doing no longer exists

Remember that any periods of disability-related absence should be ignored for the purpose of selecting an employee for redundancy. If you have worked for the same employer for two years or more you will be able to claim statutory redundancy pay. The amount will depend on your age, salary and length of service and your employer must give you a statement setting out how your redundancy pay has been calculated.

Currently you are entitled to:

- half a week's pay for each year of employment during which you were aged 21 or under
- one week's pay for each year of employment in which you were aged between 22 and 40
- one and a half week's pay for each year of employment in which you were aged 41 or over

The maximum number of years that can be taken into account is 20 and a week's pay is subject to an upper limit that is set annually.

When are dismissals not redundancies?

If you think that the real reason that you have been selected for redundancy is because of your condition or because you care for someone with Parkinson's then you may be able to make a claim for unfair dismissal and disability discrimination.

You need to seek legal advice as soon as possible, as strict time limits apply for making claims to the Employment Tribunal or the Industrial Tribunal in Northern Ireland. You can get help from your Trade Union if you are a member or from your local Citizens Advice Bureau, Law Centre or from the Disability Law Service. Contact the Labour Relations Agency in Northern Ireland. See back of book for details.

If your job still needs to be done but you are not able to do the work for any reason, including because of your disability, this is not a redundancy. If you resign or are dismissed for any reason this is not because of redundancy, even if you don't have another job to go to.

An employee whose contract is terminated by the employer because they are no longer able to do their job or a suitable alternative job, even with reasonable adjustments, is also not redundant if the work they used to do still needs to be done by another employee.

Ask for redeployment as a reasonable adjustment

If there are no reasonable adjustments that would mean you could do your current job, your employers must look for suitable alternative jobs that you can be transferred to. Remember that the job might be suitable if other reasonable adjustments are made (for example, changing hours or location, providing equipment).

It is not enough for your employer to simply let you know about internal jobs and suggest that you apply. Disabled employees who need to be redeployed as a reasonable adjustment should not have to take part in competitive interviews for vacant jobs, if they are qualified to do them, or would be with a reasonable amount of training and support.

This is redeployment as a reasonable adjustment under the Equality Act and is different to redeployment of an employee, disabled or not, who is at risk of being made redundant.

If you can't do your job, even with reasonable adjustments, and there is no other suitable job in the organisation for you, your employer can terminate your contract. This may be a fair dismissal and as you are not redundant you will not be entitled to a redundancy payment. This is because your job still needs to be done and your employer will have to find someone else to do your job.

Retiring from work

Some people with Parkinson's may start thinking about giving up work completely before reaching state retirement age. This may be because they feel that working with Parkinson's is becoming too difficult and they want to concentrate on other aspects of their life.

If you do decide to retire, it may take time to adjust to life without work. Talking to someone may help. This may be a family member, trusted friend or others who have gone through retirement. A counsellor can also help.

Ill-health retirement and Permanent Health Insurance (PHI) schemes

If you have been paying into a pension scheme you may be able to take early ill health retirement. Whether or not this is possible will depend on the terms of your pension scheme. If you retire early but are still medically fit for work, the amount you get may be lower.

If you have ill health or disability insurance you may be able to make a claim on that policy. Remember, however, that to make a claim on such a permanent ill health or PHI scheme you need to be employed. If your contract of employment is terminated, you will not be able to claim on your insurance policy. If this happens you should seek legal advice as you may have a claim for breach of contract. To make sure you are aware of all your options when getting your pension, it is advisable to talk to an independent financial adviser.

Work and caring for someone with Parkinson's

You may be working as well as caring for someone with Parkinson's. Paid work can provide financial independence and money to help with caring, a break from caring, social networks and friendships, self-esteem and a better pension, but combining your responsibilities has its own challenges. Your employment needs should be taken into account in any assessment from your local authority.

Carers and discrimination in the workplace

If you care for someone with Parkinson's you are protected from being discriminated against or harassed at work because of your link to someone with a disability, such as a long-term condition. This means that as a carer you should not be treated less favourably than another employee who isn't a carer, and should not be denied the flexibility you are legally entitled to. Any offensive language about your association with a person with Parkinson's should also not be tolerated.

Informing your employer that you are a carer

You do not have to tell your employer you are a carer but it may help if they are aware if you need to take time off to look after the person you care for. Checking your employee handbook or talking to the human resources department will also help you find out what support may be available to you at work. You might make this decision depending on whether your employer has a policy to support carers, or whether they'd be open to exploring ways to support you. Find out what's available before you approach your manager.

As a working carer, you are likely to need a range of support – such as access to a telephone to check on the person you care for. An understanding employer can make all the difference to whether or not you feel you can seek support.

Flexible working hours

You don't have the right to ask for reasonable adjustments but you may have a statutory (legal) right to ask your employer if you can work flexibly. This may mean changing your hours or working from home.

Your right to make this request will depend on your relationship to the person with Parkinson's and how long you have been working at your company. Your employer must give serious consideration to your request but they can refuse if there are good business reasons for doing so. Requests made under the statutory scheme will, if agreed, become permanent changes to your terms and conditions.

To find out more about who has the statutory right to ask for flexible working visit www.gov.uk/flexible-working

Whether or not you meet the criteria for making a statutory request for work flexibility, remember that there is nothing stopping you from making an informal request to your employer. This may also be appropriate if you need a temporary change to your terms and conditions.

Getting support

If you are a member of a trade union, ask them for help. A local, or regional, union representative may be able to negotiate with your employer on your behalf and attend meetings with you.

If you are not in a union, you have the right to have a colleague attend certain types of meeting with you.

Time off in an emergency

The Employment Rights Act 1996 allows employees to take a 'reasonable' amount of time off work to deal with an emergency involving a dependent.

A dependant could be one of the following.

- husband or wife
- partner
- child
- parent
- friend or family member who lives with you but doesn't pay rent
- someone who relies on you to care for them (for example, an elderly neighbour)

You should also find out how unpaid time off might affect your work rights, pension and working tax credit eligibility.

In the next chapter we look at the range of benefits available if you do decide to leave work or if you are out of work anyway.

****

Chapter 10

Welfare Benefits for Parkinson's Sufferers, Family and Carers

---

The benefits system is daunting at the best of times. There are so many benefits available and so many different rules and regulations. However, it is important to gain an understanding of the core benefits that may be available to those who suffer from Parkinson's and those who care for them. As a minimum, a person with Parkinson's can usually claim Attendance Allowance, Disability Living Allowance (care component) or the new Personal Independence Payment (the daily living component). Carers should check their entitlement to Carer's allowance.

The benefits described below are available in England and Wales. Benefits in Northern Ireland and Scotland largely mirror those in England, but there are some differences (such as with Council tax support). People claiming benefits in Scotland and Northern Ireland should contact the Benefit Enquiry Line in Northern Ireland/Scotland (see end of chapter).

This chapter discusses benefits generally. However, for more in-depth advice on the range of benefits available for those suffering from Parkinson's, or their carers, you should go to the Citizens Advice website or to Parkinson's UK. There is a list of useful addresses at the end of this chapter.

How to claim benefits-Qualifying for benefits

To qualify for any benefit, you will have to meet certain conditions. These vary according to the type of benefit. Some benefits depend on you having paid National Insurance contributions over a period of time, some on the amount of your weekly income and savings, and some on the practical effects of a disability.

Where to claim

The Department for Work and Pensions (DWP) is responsible for administering the state pension and benefits.

The system is organised so that:

- benefits relating to people of working age are dealt with by Jobcentre Plus offices
- the State Pension and other benefits relating to people of state-pension age are dealt with by the Pension Service
- disability benefits are dealt with by the Disability Benefits Centre
- Carer's allowance is dealt with by the Carer's Allowance Unit
- in addition, Her Majesty's Revenue and Customs (HMRC) deal with benefits relating to children, as well as tax credits.

Making a claim

You claim benefits either by filling in forms and sending them in the post, or by phoning a contact centre where an adviser will complete the form and send it to you to sign and return. Some benefits can be claimed by completing an online form on the gov.uk website.

Challenging a decision

Most people receive the benefits they are entitled to without a problem. However, if you believe your claim has been incorrectly turned down, or that you have not been awarded the right amount of benefit, you have the right to challenge the decision. Write to the office that made the decision and ask them to revise it. If they do not alter their decision, you may be able to apply to an independent appeal tribunal.

Challenging a decision can be complex, and seeking advice as soon as possible can really help. Ask your local CAB or advice centre, your local authority's welfare rights unit, or the Parkinson's UK Helpline (details in the useful resources section) .

Care and mobility benefits-Attendance Allowance, Disability Living Allowance and Personal Independence Payments

People with dementia, as anyone else, do not automatically qualify for disability benefits - tests are required to determine the level of need. For people who do qualify, these benefits provide extra help to deal with the practical effects of a disability. They are tax free, and do not depend on National Insurance contributions. Payment is not affected by the person's savings or income. A medical assessment may be required. These benefits are paid at different rates, depending on the person's needs. They can be claimed whether the person works or not, and whether they live alone, with their family or with other people.

If your care needs started after the age of 65, or you have not made a claim until then, you should claim Attendance allowance (AA) (see below). This is for help with personal care, not mobility. If you have care and/or mobility needs and are aged under 65, you should claim Personal independence payment (PIP) instead. You must be under 65 when you make your first claim.

It is important to seek advice if you are already claiming one of these benefits and your needs change. If you are already claiming Disability Living Allowance you should be transferred to PIP by 2018. You don't need to initiate the claim for PIP if you are already getting DLA - you will get an invitation to claim. However, if you don't respond to the invitation, your DLA will be stopped. People who receive PIP before they are 65 will be able to stay on it after they reach 65.

The claim forms for PIP and AA are very detailed and lengthy. There are questions about the activities that the person with dementia finds difficult or impossible to carry out, and about their need for care and supervision. You should consider the bad days as well as the good when thinking about the help needed. It is very important to get advice from a professional (including advice centre staff) on filling in the form to make sure you are giving the information that is needed.

Attendance allowance

Personal care needs might include supervision of, or help with, activities such as washing, dressing, eating, going to the toilet, turning over or settling in bed, taking medication, avoiding danger, or attending social or recreational activities. If you have a disabling condition such as Parkinson's and are over 65, you may qualify for AA at one of the following levels:

- Higher rate - if you need frequent help or prompting with personal care like washing or going to the toilet, or continual supervision to avoid danger during the day and also need help with personal care either for a prolonged period or several times during the night, or if you need watching over.

- Lower rate - if you need frequent help or prompting with personal care, or continual supervision throughout the day, or help either for a prolonged period or several times during the night, or if you need watching over.

Personal Independence Payment

PIP has daily living components and (unlike AA) also mobility components. Depending on your situation, you may qualify for either or both. If you have a disabling condition such as parkinson's and are under 65, you may qualify for the daily living component of PIP at one of the following levels:

- standard rate - if you have a limited ability to carry out daily living activities

- enhanced rate - if you have a severely limited ability to carry out daily living activities. if you have difficulties getting out and about, you may qualify for the mobility component of PIP at one of the following levels:

- standard rate - if you have limited mobility, which can include the ability to plan a journey or manage it unaided (it's not just about the ability to walk).

- enhanced rate - if you have severely limited mobility (as above).

Making a claim consists of two stages: the basic claim and the claimant questionnaire. The basic claim is made by telephone, or in writing by completing a PIP1 form. This is to establish the claim, and to ensure that you are eligible to apply.

Once the basic claim has been successfully made, a claimant questionnaire (PIP2 - How your disability affects you) will be sent to you. This is aimed at gathering more information about how your health condition or impairment affects your day-to-day life. During the basic claim stage, people who may have additional support needs, for example because of a cognitive impairment, should be contacted by the assessment providers to attend a medical assessment.

Disability living allowance

Although this benefit is being phased out for people aged 16-64, some existing claimants may still be re-assessed for it when their claim comes up for review. This is because they live in an area where PIP isn't yet being introduced for existing claimants. If this affects you, you will need to complete the form as you have in the past, referring to your care and mobility needs as they currently are. You will be re-assessed for PIP at a later date.

If you go into a care home or hospital, temporarily or permanently, get advice about how your AA, PIP or DLA might be affected.

Benefits if unable to work

The following are benefits that can be claimed if you are working but are no longer able to work:

Statutory sick pay

This is paid by employers to employees below retirement age, for up to 28 weeks in any one period of sickness. To qualify, you must earn a set amount or more each week before tax and be off work because of sickness. This benefit is paid at a flat rate and is taxable.

Employment and Support Allowance (ESA)

Employment and Support Allowance has two forms - contributory ESA (which replaced Incapacity benefit) and income-related ESA (which replaced Income support claimed on the grounds of incapacity for work). People with Incapacity benefit or Income support on the grounds of incapacity for work are being transferred to Employment and support allowance. You can still receive Income support if you qualify on grounds other than incapacity - see 'Income support' below.

Carers' needs-Carer's allowance

This benefit can be paid to carers who spend at least 35 hours per week looking after someone who is receiving DLA (care component at highest or middle rate), PIP (daily living component at either rate) or Attendance allowance (at either rate). The carer does not have to be related to, or living with, the person they provide care for.

The benefit does not depend on National Insurance contributions, but it is taxable. It gives most carers who are under State pension age a National Insurance credit each week to help protect their State Pension rights. Carers must be over 16 when they first claim. In some cases, the person being cared for could lose some of their means-tested benefits if Carer's Allowance is paid, so it is important to seek advice before making a claim.

Carers are not eligible for Carer's Allowance if they earn more than a limited amount each week after the deduction of allowable expenses (such as Income tax and pension contributions), if they are in full-time education, or if they are receiving more than a specified amount from certain other pensions or benefits.

People entitled to Carer's Allowance may be entitled to additional amounts in other benefits they are claiming, such as Income Support or Pension Credit. This may be the case even for those who are entitled to Carer's Allowance but cannot receive the payments because they are already receiving certain other pensions or benefits. That is, if the person qualifies for Carers Allowance but receives an 'overlapping benefit' - where you are eligible for different benefits but can only receive one at any one time. If you are a carer and are unsure about your entitlement, you should seek advice from Carers UK.

Depending on their income, a carer may be able to claim a higher rate of benefit if their spouse or partner is dependent on them financially. If a carer has dependent children, they may also be able to claim Child Tax Credit.

Retirement-The Pension Service
DWP set up the Pension Service to deal with the State pension and other pension-related benefits. If you have reached, or are nearing, State pension age, the Pension Service will write to you and give you a phone number to call for information. Your queries will usually be

dealt with over the phone or by post, but the service can arrange for someone to visit you at home, if necessary.

State pension

A State pension is paid to people who reach State pension age if they have made sufficient National Insurance Contributions. It is taxable. The State pension age for men is currently 65. The State pension age for women born on or before 5 April 1950 is 60. The pension age for men and women is gradually rising so that by 2020 it will be 66. After that it will rise to 68 for both men and women.

People who do not have sufficient contributions may receive a reduced State pension or no pension at all. Under the previous rules, women and widowed people, divorced people, civil partners and same sex spouses who did not have sufficient contributions of their own were able to claim on the contributions of their partner or former partner. From April 2016 this will no longer be possible.

People may also qualify for extra pension for a number of reasons. People over 80 who do not qualify for a State pension or full State Pension may be eligible for an over-80s pension, which does not depend on National Insurance Contributions.

You can claim your pension if you are still working. However, if you want to, you can defer your pension and then draw a higher weekly pension when you do claim it.

If you are entitled to a State Pension, the Pension Service should contact you about four months before you reach State Pension age. If you have not heard anything three months before reaching State

Pension age, contact your social security office or the Pension Service claims line.

There is going to be a new State pension from April 2016, but only for people who reach State pension age on or after April 2016. The basic pension will be set at a higher level for these new retirees, but they will need a longer National insurance record of their own, and certain other pension additions will be phased out.

If you are below State pension age but unable to work, you may be able to protect your State Pension rights by getting National insurance contribution credits. These are automatically given to people receiving certain benefits, such as Incapacity Benefit, Employment and Support allowance and Carer's Allowance.

Alternatively, carers who do not receive these benefits may be able to protect their rights through a weekly carers credit to build up their State Pension entitlement. This scheme replaces the Home Responsibilities Protection Scheme and may make a considerable difference to your State pension. Previous protection built up under the Home Responsibilities Protection Scheme will be incorporated into the new system. If you think you may be eligible, seek advice.

Pension credit

If you are unable to claim the State Pension, or it is not enough for you to live on, you may be entitled to claim other benefits, such as Pension Credit. The age at which men and women are eligible to claim Pension Credit will increase in line with the changes in the State Pension age for women (see 'State Pension' above). Pension Credit is a means-tested benefit. It has two parts: Guarantee Credit and Savings Credit. Guarantee Pension Credit works by topping up a person's income if they are on a low income. Savings Credit is extra money for people aged 65 and over who have an income level above the basic retirement pension level, or who have savings or investments. No new claims for Savings Credit will be taken from April 2016, but people who already receive it will continue to do so.

Some people are entitled to both the Guarantee and Savings Credits, while others are entitled to one or the other. People eligible for Pension Credit may also qualify for other benefits such as help with housing costs, and NHS costs.

Help for people on a low income-Income Support

Income Support is a means-tested benefit to help people with basic living expenses who have not reached the qualifying age for Pension Credit and who are not required to be available for work, such as carers. There are strict criteria for people who qualify for Income support.

You may be able to claim Income Support if you have a low income and limited savings, or limited joint savings with a partner. Whether or not you qualify may depend on the number of hours you and any partner work each week. Income support can be paid in full or as a top up to other pensions and income. If you have a partner, you must claim Income support together.

Income Support does not depend on National Insurance contributions, but savings and income (including income from most benefits) will be taken into account. Income from AA, DLA and PIP will be ignored when calculating weekly income, but savings over a certain amount usually mean you cannot receive Income sSpport. The amount of Income Support paid varies according to age, existing income and savings, and entitlement to any available premiums.

Premiums are awarded to people receiving certain disability benefits and carers receiving the Carer's Allowance, for example, so it is important to seek advice.

If you are a homeowner, you may receive help with mortgage interest payments, interest payments on loans for certain repairs and improvements, ground rent and some service charges. This will depend on the circumstances of those living in your home. You may not qualify for immediate help with your housing costs.

You can no longer claim Income Support if you cannot work because you have a disability or illness. You should claim ESA instead.

Cold weather and winter fuel payments

Cold weather payments are paid if the average temperature in your area falls or is forecast to fall to freezing point or below for seven consecutive days. These payments are made automatically to people receiving some means-tested benefits including Pension credit and Income support.

If you are of eligible age, you will normally qualify for a winter fuel payment to help with the cost of fuel. The age at which people receive a winter fuel payment is rising because it is linked to the

State Pension age for women, which is also increasing (see 'State Pension' above).

People over 80 may be eligible for more money. Many people living in care homes are not eligible for this payment. This benefit is not means-tested or taxable, and will not affect any other benefits you are claiming. For more information, or to apply, contact the Winter fuel payment helpline.

Help with housing costs

If you receive Income Support, income-related Employment and Support Allowance, Income-Related Jobseeker's allowance or Guarantee Credit, you may qualify for help with your rent, Council tax and NHS costs. You may also be eligible to apply for help with your rent and Council Tax if you are on a low income, such as low wages or Savings Credit.

Support for mortgage interest

You may get help paying some of your mortgage interest, if you are entitled to Income Support, Income-Related ESA, income-based Jobseeker's Allowance, or Pension Guarantee Credit (and Universal credit when eventually introduced).

Housing benefit

Housing benefit is a benefit to help pay for rent. It is assessed and paid for by local councils. The amount of benefit paid will normally depend on the person's income and savings, and the rent being charged. You may not be eligible for Housing benefit if you have savings over a set amount.

People renting from a private landlord usually have their Housing Benefit limited to what is known as the Local Housing Allowance. Local Housing Allowance rates can be found on local authority websites. In some instances, a room for a carer can be included in the amounts.

Similar provisions now also apply to people of working age only, living in social sector housing. The under-occupancy size criteria (often referred to as the bedroom tax) means that, if it is considered that you have too many bedrooms, the amount of your rent eligible for housing benefit will be cut by 14% (for one bedroom too many) or 25% (for two or more bedrooms too many).

If you live with a partner, only one of you should apply for Housing Benefit. However, your income and savings will be considered jointly and other adults living with you will affect the amount of Housing Benefit you can receive. Housing benefit does not depend on National Insurance Contributions and is tax free. It can be claimed at the same time as Income Support, Income-Based Jobseeker's Allowance, Income-Related ESA or Pension Credit.

A claim form for Housing Benefit is included in the application packs for means-tested benefits.If you are not applying for another benefit you can ask the local authority for an application form.

Help with Council Tax

The Council Tax is set by local authorities to pay for the services they provide. The amount of Council Tax support that a person or couple is eligible for depends on income and savings, and the amount of Council Tax due. People under pension age may be asked to pay a contribution to the tax even if on a low income.

Help with NHS costs-NHS benefits

People receiving Income Support, Income-Based Jobseeker's Allowance, Pension Credit, Working Tax Credit (a payment that you may qualify for if you work but are on a low income) or income-related ESA might receive help with:

- free prescriptions (prescriptions are also free for anyone aged 60 and over)
- free dental treatment from NHS dentists
- free sight tests and vouchers towards the cost of glasses - sight tests are also free for anyone aged 60 and over
- help with hospital travel costs for NHS treatment and free appliances for outpatients or day patients.

NHS hearing aids are prescribed by an NHS consultant to anyone needing them on free loan. They are fitted, serviced and supplied with batteries free of charge.

NHS low income scheme

If you do not receive any of the above benefits but are on a low income and have savings below the limit, you can apply for help towards NHS health costs. The amount of financial help you receive will depend on your savings and income.

You need to complete form HC1, which you can get from Jobcentre Plus offices and NHS hospitals. Some GPs, dentists and opticians may also stock them. If you live in a care home you can apply on a special short form called HC1(SC). Ask the care home manager or a carer for this form or use the HC1 form. For more information on help with NHS costs, see the booklet HC11 Help with health costs, available from any of the above sources or search for 'HC11' on the Department of Health website.

Special notes

Benefits in hospital

Benefits may be affected if either a carer or a person with dementia goes into an NHS hospital for more than a short stay. In this case, it is important to seek advice and inform the local social security office, Jobcentre Plus office, Pension Centre or DWP Disability and Carers Service as appropriate.

Useful organisations for benefits advice

Age UK
Tavis House
1-6 Tavistock Square
London WC1H 9NA
T 0800 169 6565 (advice line)
E contact@ageuk.org.uk
W www.ageuk.org.uk

Wales - Age Cymru
T 08000 223 444 (advice line)
E enquiries@agecymru.org.uk
W www.agecymru.org.uk

Northern Ireland - Age NI

T 0808 808 7575 (advice line)

E info@ageni.org

W www.ageuk.org.uk/northern-ireland

Provides information and advice for older people in the UK.

Carers UK

20 Great Dover Street

London SE1 4LX

T 0808 808 7777 (advice line) Monday -

Friday 10am-4pm

E advice@carersuk.org

W www.carersuk.org

Citizens Advice Bureau (CAB)

Various locations

W www.citizensadvice.org.uk

www.adviceguide.org.uk

(online information resource)

Your local CAB can provide information and advice in confidence or point you in the right direction to further sources of support. Trained CAB advisers can offer information on benefits in a way that is easy to understand. To find your nearest CAB, look in the phone book, ask at your local library or look on the website (above). Opening times vary.

Department of Health

Richmond House

79 Whitehall

London SW1A 2NS
T 020 7210 4850 (8.30am-5.30pm weekdays)
020 7210 5025 (textphone)
E use the enquiry form on the website (see below)
W www.dh.gov.uk

The government department responsible for health, social care, and the National Health Service (NHS). Provides a range of information and literature, including help with NHS costs.

Department for Work and Pensions (DWP)
W www.gov.uk

The government department responsible for employment and social security. The gov.uk website gives details of the various benefits and how to claim them, as well as information on pensions and pension credits. Claim forms are available to download.

Disability Benefits Centre
W www.gov.uk/disability-benefits-helpline

Personal Independence Payment (PIP)
T 0345 850 3322
Textphone: 0345 601 6677
Monday to Friday, 8am-6pm

Personal Independence Payment
(New claims only)
T 0800 917 2222
Textphone: 0800 917 7777
Monday to Friday, 8am-6pm

Disability Living Allowance
T 0345 712 3456
Textphone: 0345 722 4433
Monday to Friday, 8am-6pm

Attendance Allowance (also for DLA claimants who are 65+)
T 0345 605 6055
Textphone: 0345 604 5312
Monday to Friday, 8am-6pm

Winter Fuel Payments Helpline
T 0845 915 1515 (8.30am-4.30pm weekdays)
W www.gov.uk/winter-fuel-payment

State Pension and Pension Credit enquiries
T 0345 60 60 265 (8am-6pm weekdays)
State pension claim line
T 0800 731 7898 (8am-6pm weekdays)
W www.gov.uk/state-pension

NHS Help with health costs advice line
T 0300 330 1343

Provides NHS patients with information about entitlements to prescription charge exemptions and the requirements to qualify for exemptions.

Northern Ireland - Benefit Enquiry Line
T 0800 220 674 (9am-5pm weekdays except Thursday; 10am-5pm Thursday)
028 9031 1092 (textphone, 9am-5pm weekdays)

Provides advice and information on Attendance allowance, Disability living allowance, Personal independence payments, Carer's allowance and Carer's credit.

Welfare benefits Scotland

https://www.citizensadvice.org.uk/scotland/benefits

****

Chapter 11

Living and Coping with Parkinson's Disease-General Advice

When a person first receives a diagnosis of Parkinson's disease, it can be very stressful and also confusing, both for the individual and family and friends. It is crucial, at the outset, that advice and information is available.

One of the most important factors in the life of someone with Parkinson's disease, particularly someone who has been newly diagnosed, is that of ongoing support. There is a lot of support out there, not least the umbrella groups such as Parkinson's UK who can be contacted on 0808 800 0303 e mail hello@parkinsons.org.uk or online at www. parkinsons.org.uk.

In addition, there are Parkinson's disease nurse specialists who are community based or based in a hospital. Their numbers have expanded over the years although there is not yet one in every area. They are registered nurses who have specialised in the area of Parkinson's disease and they have broad experience in neurology or the care of elderly people. Their work involves assessing individual care needs, enhancing and promoting quality of life and preventing, or at least minimising the complications associated with Parkinson's disease. Typical complications can include problems with mobility, urinary problems, depression, and the side effects of medication.

Therapies for Parkinson's disease

Parkinson's disease can interfere, to a greater or lesser extent, with many day-to-day activities. The aim of therapies is to ease these difficulties by helping you to learn the knowledge and skills that you will need to continue with a normal life. There are three main therapies available, physiotherapy, occupational therapy and speech and language therapy.

Physiotherapy

A physiotherapist will assess your needs by looking at the difficulties that you have with movement and general mobility. The aim of the physiotherapist is to help you achieve the greatest level of activity possible. They will teach you how to manage the physical problems associated with Parkinson's disease.

Beware of those who call themselves physiotherapists. A Qualified physiotherapist will be a member of the Chartered Society of Physiotherapists. Each person will specialise in a different area of physiotherapy, as with most other professions and not all physiotherapists have the required expertise in neurological disorders. Physiotherapists interested in neurological disorders will be senior practitioners and will often be termed neurophysiotherapists.

Physiotherapy will help you move more normally and with less effort. Physiotherapy is not about routine exercise, as has already been outlined in this book, but about learning skills and techniques to assist you with coping with problems that arise with the onset and development of the disease. Certain basic tasks, which you have found easy all your life, such as tying a tie or doing up your shoelaces can become a chore when you have Parkinson's. Physiotherapy will teach you certain techniques and provide learning strategies, such as talking through a task while doing it or relying on visual targets to improve performance. These approaches are known as cueing.

Stiffness and poor posture also comes with Parkinson's. Muscles and joints will stiffen up over time making it increasingly harder to walk and relax. Physiotherapists can help to relieve this muscle and joint stiffness. Physiotherapists can also advise you about appropriate exercises that will help you, such as swimming or the Alexander technique.

Occupational therapy

Occupational therapists will assist you in those daily aspects of life that have become increasingly more difficult, such as looking after yourself and others, and also with work and leisure. It can also be difficult for you to travel where you want, because of mobility problems. Occupational therapists will work with you to improve your life by identifying areas of particular difficulty and devising a programme specifically for you to help you overcome these problems.

A qualified occupational therapist will be state registered and have a degree (BSc (Hons) OT) or diploma (DipCot). As with physiotherapists occupational therapists specialise in different areas. These occupational therapists who have specialised in neurological disorders might be members of NANOT (National Association of Neurological OT's) or have done some further specialised training after initially qualifying as an occupational therapist.

Speech and language therapists

A speech and language therapist will work with Parkinson's sufferers and also, where necessary, with family or carers. They will identify where the difficulties impact on lifestyle, such as using the telephone or when conversing in shops or at work. Therapy will include exercises that work on improving voice loudness and intelligibility of speech generally. Communication can be affected by the types of swallowing difficulties encountered by people with Parkinson's, which include difficulties controlling saliva, difficulty chewing harder foods and problems with swallowing generally. Some may experience coughing or choking episodes while eating. A speech and language therapist will assess swallowing problems and provide advice on the easiest food and drinks and also the safest approach to eating and drinking. It is highly advisable to see a therapist as soon as possible after your initial diagnosis of Parkinson's. Your family doctor or consultant will usually make the referral to see a therapist

Driving and Parkinson's

A diagnosis of Parkinson's does not always mean that you will have to cease driving. However, you must by law inform the Driver and Vehicle Licensing Agency (DVLA). You can continue to drive after informing the DVLA until they inform you other wise. If you or your family or friends have any concerns, however, you should stop driving and discuss the matter with your doctor.

The DVLA assesses each case individually and may issue either a restricted licence, (restricted to a number of years or to a vehicle with adaptations) or an unrestricted licence. Both of these will allow you to continue driving once you have been diagnosed with Parkinson's. However, the DVLA can also decide that you should not be allowed to drive for a specified period. If you are not happy with the DVLA's decision then you can appeal asking them to reconsider or you can appeal in a magistrate's court.

When you contact the DVLA, you will need to complete two forms, PK1 'Medical in confidence' available from the DirectGov website and a shorter medical questionnaire detailing your symptoms and you may be required to undergo further medical assessment and possibly retake the practical part of the driving test. Medicals and driving tests are free to those newly diagnosed with Parkinson's. A more detailed booklet is available from www.parkinsons.org.uk.

Parkinson's medication and driving

The side effects that some people might experience from their medication can affect driving. Dopamine agonists can cause drowsiness, sometime severe. You need to be aware of this and consult the literature about side effects provided with your medication. You can also get advice from your doctor.

Mobility centres and driving assessment.

Mobility centres provide information and advice on driving for any person who is disabled and uses a car, either as a driver or a passenger. They will also offer assessments on your ability to drive a vehicle. There are a number of mobility centres in the UK, again information can be obtained from the DVLA website or from www.parkinsons.org.uk.

Priority parking and the Blue Badge Scheme

You may qualify for parking concessions through the Blue Badge Scheme if you have a severe disability and also qualify for the higher rate of the mobility component of the Disability Living Allowance (see chapter on benefits). The Blue Badge Scheme enables people who have certain disabilities to park closer to shops and the services that they need to get to. The badge applies whether they are driver or passenger in a vehicle. More information can be obtained from the DirectGov website www.directgov.co.uk. In addition to the above, if you are disabled and qualify for DLA or the War Pensioners Mobility Supplement you may also be eligible for a car tax exemption.

Car insurance and Parkinson's

If you have been diagnosed with Parkinson's you should inform your car insurance company as any changes in your health may affect your ability to drive and render your policy invalid. It is also an offence under the Road Traffic Act not to inform your insurer of changes of circumstances.

You must also inform your insurers about any adaptations to your vehicle. Insurers will want to know about any disabilities or health problems, particularly if there have been any restrictions imposed on your licence. Insurers are not allowed to refuse insurance to disabled drivers unless they can justify it. Any insurance premium has to be based on a reasonable assessment of risk.

If you feel that an insurer has behaved unreasonably or has not acted within the remit of the Equality Act 2010 (see Parkinson's and employment) you should complain directly to the insurer. If the response of the Insurer is not satisfactory then you should go to the Financial Services Ombudsman (address at the back of the book).

Adaptations to vehicles for drivers with Parkinson's

If you have Parkinson's and it is impacting on your driving comfort and safety, then you can get your vehicle adapted to suit your particular condition. There are motoring accessories available for people with upper or lower body disabilities or both, which include:

- Hand controls to operate the accelerator or break
- Aids to help you turn the steering wheel with greater ease
- Accessories to help you get in and out of your vehicle such as cushions, covers and support
- Adapted mirrors for greater vision
- Different types of seat belts and harnesses
- Lifts and wheelchair hoists.

This list is not exclusive there are a number of adaptations which would be recommended at the time of fitting.

Dropped kerbs

A dropped kerb can make it easier to access your vehicle. For this you would normally apply to your local county council (or your local authority who can advise). More information is available on the DirectGov website.

****

Chapter 12

People who care for Parkinson's Sufferer's

Definition of a carer

We have all heard of the word "carer". This denotes a number of things. A carer can be someone who looks after their mother or father or looks after someone else in the family or a friend in an unpaid capacity. A carer is quite different to a home help.

Someone who is in the position of a carer for a person who has been diagnosed with Parkinson's can claim benefits in certain circumstances, access help and support from social services and also receive priority support from local health services. Carer's benefits are outlined in the chapter on welfare benefits.

Providing care to a person with Parkinson's

As the symptoms associated with Parkinson's will change over time, the nature of the care that is provided will also, of necessity, change with that person's needs. For example, in the early stages of Parkinson's the level of care needed may be minimal. It is at this early stage that it is important to gather as much information as you possibly can about the condition so you can become acquainted with the possible future needs of the person. You can gather information from a number of sources, the Internet, for example from Parkinson's UK www.parkinsons.org.uk or from medical and social services providers.

Many people with Parkinson's stay independent for years after their initial diagnosis and won't really need a lot of care. It is important during this time to display a positive attitude which can be of great benefit to your partner or relative/friend and can make a significant difference to how they cope with Parkinson's. There are a number of ways that you as a carer can assist, such as encouraging them to lead as active and normal a life as is possible under the circumstances and allowing them to do as much for themselves as possible.

If you feel that you need further training and advice in this area there are a number of courses, and informal groupings, available for carer's which explore the issues involved and allow you to meet other people in the same circumstances. There are useful contacts listed at the end of this chapter and at the back of the book.

Talking to health professionals

Your GP will be the first person you should talk to about your caring responsibilities. Carer's are given special consideration because of their role and the pressure that comes with that role. It always helps to compile a list of your needs and of the concerns that you wish to discuss with your doctor. Again, Parkinson's UK has useful information relating to discussing things with your doctor.

Following discussions with your GP, he/she will then, through the primary care team provide support and advice and:

- Arrange home visits to you or the person that you care for
- Arrange appointments for you and the person that you care for at the same time

- Supply repeat prescriptions to be delivered to your local pharmacy
- Put you in touch with other sources of support and advice such as other voluntary advice agencies
- Provide any letters of support that may be required for benefit departments or other agencies, such as the Blue Badge Scheme.

The Carer's Register

A carer's register is a database compiled by (some) surgeries that will enable staff to identify carer's and also those in receipt of care. The register is used to help get the right services at the right time, provide clear information about other relevant services and receive up-to-date information about events for carer's. In addition, the register will ensure that appointments are offered at appropriate times and that outpatient appointments and letters make clear that the person is a carer.

Time off from caring

Time of from caring is known as a 'Respite Break'. Time off from caring responsibilities is very important. Taking a break can help alleviate the anxieties and depression that accompany the role of carer. Respite breaks don't always mean that you have to go away somewhere, they can be given in a variety of ways, such as a social services care worker taking over for a while, or someone from a charity such as Crossroads Care (address at the back of the book) coming to the home regularly to care for the person with Parkinson's. In addition, the person that you care for can spend some time at a day centre or can spend short periods in a care home. All of this will depend on the circumstances at the time.

Carer's assessments

The local authority in your area has responsibility for arranging services that can help you take a break from caring. This will be achieved through a carer's assessment. Social services then use the assessment to decide what services to provide. You would normally initiate the assessment by visiting the social services department of the local council and asking for an assessment for the person that you care for and also for yourself as the carer.

The social services department will also carry out a financial assessment, which may mean that either you or the person being cared for will be responsible for all or some of the services provided. The decision to charge will be according to means.

Carers and employment rights

We discussed carers rights in chapter ten, dealing with rights whilst in employment. If you are in the position where you are caring for someone with Parkinson's and also working at the same time, you may find that the pressure on you as a person increases significantly. Carer's have statutory rights at work that can help reduce this pressure and also help to meet other needs. Employers also may be able to offer additional flexibility through their own policies and procedures.

Telling your employer about your role as a carer

There is no legal obligation to inform your employer about your role as carer. If you decide to tell your employer then make sure that you are fully aware of your statutory rights. You can find detailed information about your rights and employer's responsibilities from Carers UK www.carersuk.org and DirectGov.

Statutory rights for carer's

The main law protecting carer's in the workplace is the Work and Families Act 2006 and the Employment Rights Act 1996, which give working carer's rights to help them manage work and caring. This includes the right to request flexible work and leave entitlement. In Northern Ireland they are called the Work and Families (Northern Ireland) Order 2006 and the Employment Rights (Northern Ireland) Order 2006. Your employment status can affect your entitlement to statutory rights. If you are self-employed, on a short term contract or employed through an agency you may not be covered by these rights. If this applies to you, contact ACAS on 08457 47 47 47 for further advice.

Your employer may already have procedures in place to support carer's. This will usually be within the staff handbook or the intranet. The size and nature of the employer will determine whether or not they have publicized these rights. The public sector or large private sector employers are usually better at doing this.

As a working carer, you are likely to need a range of support, from access to a telephone to leave arrangements that work around the hospital visits etc of the person with Parkinson's.

You have a right to a ' reasonable' amount of time off work to deal with an emergency involving a dependant, such as a disruption or breakdown in care arrangements, a dependant falling ill or time to make better long term arrangements for a dependant. The right also includes some protection from victimisation or dismissal when you take time off. It is at the employer's discretion whether the leave is paid or unpaid.

Useful websites for carers to gain further information about the role of a carer and rights and responsibilities

Carers Direct www.nhs/carersdirect

Carers direct gives information and advice to carers

Care Directions www.caredirections.co.uk

Care Directions gives advice and information on health and care issues for older people

Carers Federation www.carersfederation.co.uk

The Carers Federation provides support for carers and for others with medical and mental health issues.

Carers UK www.carersuk.org

Carers UK is the main voice of carers in the UK providing advice and information and also campaigning on behalf of carers.

Crossroads care www.crossroads.org.uk

Crossroads provides support for carers and those being cared for.

Disabled Living Foundation www.dlf.org.uk
The Disabled Living foundation is a charity that provides advice about disability aids.

Employers for carers www.employersforcarers.org
Employers for carers provides practical advice for employers concerning the support of carers in their workforce.

Relate www.relate.org.uk
Relate provides relationship counselling and support services.

Relatives and residents association www.relres.org
The Relatives and Residents association provides advice and information on care homes and support for those with emotional concerns.

The Outsiders www.outsiders.org.uk The Outsiders is a social and peer support network of disabled people, offering advice for people who have concerns about sexual or personal relationships.

The Princess Royal Trust for Carers www.carers.org
The Princess royal trust offers information and support for carers.

Young Carers Initiative www.youngcarer.com
The Young Carers Initiative offers advice and support to young carers and their families.

****

Useful Addresses

Ability Net Central England
Freephone: 0800 269545
Web: www.abilitynet.org.uk

Information on specialist assistive technology to help people with
Any disability to use a computer.

Advisory, Conciliation and Arbitration Service (ACAS)
Helpline 0300 123 1100
www.acas.org.uk

Provides information to both employers and employees seeking
information on employment rights and obligations.

British Association / College of Occupational Therapists
106-114 Borough High Street
London
SE1 1LB
Tel:020 7357 6480 or
020 7450 2330
www.cot.org.uk

Information about all aspects of Occupational
Therapy. An S.A.E. requested.

Carers UK
20 Great Dover Street
London

SE1 4LX
Tel: 020 7378 4 999
Carers' line: 0808 808 7777
www.carersuk.org

Offers information and support to all people
Who are unpaid carers, looking after others
With medical or other problems.

Chartered Society of Physiotherapy
14 Bedford Row
London
WC1R 4ED
Tel:020 7306 6666
www.csp.org.uk
Information about all aspects of physiotherapy.

Citizens Advice Bureaux
(National Association of CABs)
Citizens Advice
3rd Floor North
200 Aldersgate Street
London
EC1A 4HD
www.citizensadvice.org.uk

- for England call 03444 111 444
- for Wales call 03444 77 20 20
- TextRelay users should call 03444 111 445

HQ of national charity offering a wide variety of practical and legal advice. Network of local branches throughout the UK listed in phone books and Yellow Pages under Counselling and Advice.

Crossroads Caring for Carers
10 Regent Place
Rugby
Warwickshire
CV21 2PN
Helpline: 0845 450 0350
www.crossroads.org.uk

Supports and delivers high-quality service for Carers and people with care needs via its local branches.

Disability Law Service
Tel: 020 7791 9800
www.dls.org.uk

This organisation provides specialist legal advice for disabled people, their families and carers.

Disability Action (Northern Ireland)
Tel: 028 9029 7880
www.disabilityaction.org

This organisation works to ensure that people with disabilities attain their full rights as citizens, by supporting inclusion, influencing government policy and changing attitudes in partnership with disabled people.

Disabled Living Foundation

Helpline: 0300 999 0004

www.dlf.org.uk

Provides information to disabled and elderly people On all kinds of equipment in order to promote their independence and quality of life.

Disability Rights UK

Ground Floor

CAN Mezzanine

49-51 East Rd

London

N1 6AH

Tel: 020 7250 8181

www. disabilityrightsuk.org

Campaigns to improve the rights and care of disabled people. Sells special key to access locked disabled toilets.

DVLA

Driver and Vehicle Licensing Agency

Swansea

Driving Licence Enquiries
DVLA
Swansea
SA99 1BU

**Vehicle Registration and
Tax Enquiries**
DVLA

Swansea
SA99 1AR

Drivers Medical Enquiries
DVLA
Swansea
SA99 1TU

**Drivers Customer
Services**
Correspondence Team
DVLA
Swansea
SA6 7JL

Telephone	**General Enquiries:** 0300 790 6801 **Vehicle Registration and Tax:** 0300 790 6802 **Driver Check Service:** 09061 393 837 **Driver's Medical Enquiries (car or motorcycle):** 0300 790 6806 **Driver's Medical Enquiries (bus, coach or lorry):** 0300 790 6807

Provides information about Medical conditions, driving licences, learning to drive, entitlement to drive

European Parkinson's Disease Association
(EPDA)
1 Cobden Road
Sevenoaks
Kent
TN13 3UB
United Kingdom
e-mail: info@epda.eu.com

Umbrella body for network of international Parkinson's disease groups, campaigning on behalf of all suffers. Information leaflets on request. An S.A.E. requested.

Institute for Complementary and Natural Medicine
Can- Mezzanine
32-36 Loman Street
London
SE1 0EH
Tel: 0207 922 7980
www.icnm.org.uk

Umbrella group for complementary medicine organisation. Offers information, safe choice to Public.

Leonard Cheshire Disability
66 South Lambeth Road
London
SW8 1RL
Tel: 020 3242 0200
www.lcdisability.org
Email: info@lcdisability.org
Contact Customer Helpline on 0808 808 2236
email customerhelpline@lcdisability.org

National offices

Leonard Cheshire Disability Scotland
Murrayburgh House
17 Corstorphine Road
Edinburgh

EH12 6DD
Tel: 0131 346 9040
Fax: 0131 346 9050
email: scotlandoffice@LCDisability.org

Leonard Cheshire Disability Wales
Leonard Cheshire Disability Wales
Llanhennock Lodge
Llanhennock
Nr Caerleon
NP18 1LT
Tel: 01633 422583
Email: walesoffice@leonardcheshire.org

Leonard Cheshire Disability Northern Ireland
5 Boucher Plaza
4-6 Boucher Road
Belfast
BT12 6HR
Tel: 028 9024 6247
Fax: 028 9024 6395
email: northernirelandoffice@LCDisability.org

Offers care, support and a wide range of Information for disabled people aged between 18 and 65 years in the UK and worldwide to encourage independent living. Has respite and residential homes; offers holidays and rehabilitation.

Motability
Tel: 0300 456 4566
www.motability.co.uk

Helps drivers with disabilities to access specialist Cars and funding
with Motability car schemes.

National Institute for Health and Clinical Excellence (NICE)
Emailnice@nice.org.uk
Telephone+44 (0)300 323 0140

Provides national guidance on the Promotion of good health and
treatment of ill-health. Patient information leaflets are available for
each piece of guidance issued.

NHS Direct
www.nhsdirect.nhs.uk

Parkinson's UK
Hepline: 0808 800 0303
Tel: 020 7931 8080
Fax: 020 7233 9908
www.parkinsons.org.uk
Email: hello@parkinsons.org.uk

Northern Ireland office
Parkinson's UK Northern Ireland
Wellington Park Business Centre
3 Wellington Park

Malone Road
Belfast BT9 6DJ
Phone: 028 9092 3370
Email: northernireland@parkinsons.org.uk

Scotland office
Parkinson's UK Scotland
Suite 1-14
King James VI Business Centre
Riverview Business Park
Friarton Road
Perth
PH2 8DY - view map
Phone: 0344 225 3724
Email: scotland@parkinsons.org.uk
More about our work in Scotland

Wales office
Parkinson's UK Wales/Cymru
Maritime Offices
Woodland Terrace
Maesycoed
Pontypridd CF37 1DZ
Phone: 0844 225 3784
Email: wales@parkinsons.org.uk

Offers information and support via its local groups Has nurse specialists and welfare department, And funds research into Parkinson's disease.

Patients' Association
PO Box 935
Harrow
Middlesex
HA1 3YJ
Helpline: 0208 423 8999
www.patients-association.org.uk
Email: helpline@patients-association.com

Provides advice on patients' rights, leaflets and a directory of self-help groups.

Royal College of Speech and Language
Therapy
2 White Hart Yard
London
SE1 1NX
Tel: 020 7378 1200
www.rcslt.org

Information about all aspects of speech and language therapy.

YPN (Younger Parkinson's Network)
National helpline : 0808 800 0303

The young-onset self-help group of Parkinson's UK and is designed really for those of working age. There are around 1,300 members of YPN , many of them in their early 20s and 30s. Has a magazine, local meetings and conference every 2 years.
Parkinson's UK Support Group

www.parkinson.org.uk
0808 800 0303

David Rayner Centre
120 Cambridge Road
Great Shelford
Cambridege
CB22 5JT
Tel: 01223 840105
www.parkinsons.org.uk

Network of local groups bringing people with Parkinson's and their families together for support and help.

Parkinson's Home Care
Helping Hand Homecare
Arrow House
8-9 Church Street
Alcester
Warwickshire
B49 5AJ
Free phone: 0843 777 0026
www.helpinghandscare.co.uk

Specific Information for drivers
Driving and Parkinson's
Association of British Insurers (ABI) www.abi.org.uk

The ABI will assist you with any complaints that you may have about insurers

Department for Transport www.dft.gov.uk

The DFT aims to ensure that provisions for all motorists are acceptable, accessible and affordable.

Disability Alliance www.disability alliance.org

The Disability Alliance provides advice on benefits and services for people with disabilities.

Disabled Living Foundation www.dlf.org.uk

As above provides advice and information.

DVLA (Driver and Vehicle Licensing Agency) www.dvla.gov.uk

The DVLA will provide advice and information on all aspects of driving.

Mobilise www.mobilise.info

Mobilise provides help and support to disabled drivers and passengers.

Motability www.motability.co.uk
Motability helps to keep disabled drivers on the road.

****

Appendix 1
Sample medication log

As mentioned earlier in the chapter on finding and dealing with doctors and specialists, it is very important to keep a log of the medications that you take and when you take them, plus also the types of symptoms that you are experiencing. The below is an example which might help you.

Medication

Date	Time	Type and dosage	Symptoms/moods	Next dose

24 Hour record of symptoms

Date_____

Time	Medication dosage	Symptoms/moods
6am		
8am		
10am		
12noon		
2pm		
4pm		
6pm		
8pm		
10pm		

12am		
2am		
4am		

The purpose of the logs on the previous page is to ensure that you have an accurate record of what exactly is happening to you in order that both your doctor and anyone who interacts with you on a professional level understands and knows what is going on. As stated, it is likely that your doctor will have an accurate record, as this is their job, but others who deal with you may not.

****

Index

****

Emerald Imprint

Other titles in the Emerald Series:

Law
Guide to Bankruptcy
Conducting Your Own Court case
Guide to Consumer law
Creating a Will
Guide to Family Law
Guide to Employment Law
Guide to European Union Law
Guide to Health and Safety Law
Guide to Criminal Law
Guide to Landlord and Tenant Law
Guide to the English Legal System
Guide to Housing Law
Guide to Marriage and Divorce
Guide to The Civil Partnerships Act
Guide to The Law of Contract
The Path to Justice
You and Your Legal Rights
The Debt Collecting Merry Go Round
Powers of Attorney

Health
Guide to Combating Child Obesity
Asthma Begins at Home
Explaining Bipolar Disorder

The Ultimate Nutrition Guide for Cancer Sufferers and Their Friends and Family
The Ultimate Nutrition Guide for Osteoporosis Sufferers
The Sea Medicine Chest
Natures Aspirin

Music
How to Survive and Succeed in the Music Industry

General
A Practical Guide to Obtaining probate
A Practical Guide to Residential Conveyancing
Writing The Perfect CV
Keeping Books and Accounts-A Small Business Guide
Business Start Up-A Guide for New Business
Finding Asperger Syndrome in the Family-A Book of Answers
Writing Your Autobiography
Being a professional Writer

For details of the above titles published by Emerald go to:

www.straightforwardco.co.uk